The Cleveland Clinic Guide to

DIABETES

Also in *The Cleveland Clinic Guide* Series

The Cleveland Clinic Guide to Arthritis
The Cleveland Clinic Guide to Heart Attacks
The Cleveland Clinic Guide to Heart Failure
The Cleveland Clinic Guide to Infertility
The Cleveland Clinic Guide to Liver Disorders
The Cleveland Clinic Guide to Menopause
The Cleveland Clinic Guide to Prostate Cancer
The Cleveland Clinic Guide to Sleep Disorders
The Cleveland Clinic Guide to Thyroid Disorders

The Cleveland Clinic Guide to

DIABETES

S. Sethu Reddy, MD, MBA

KAPLAN

PUBLISHING

New York

© 2009 Kaplan Publishing

Published by Kaplan Publishing, a division of Kaplan, Inc.
1 Liberty Plaza, 24th Floor
New York, NY 10006

Printed in the United States of America

10 9 8 7 6 5 4 3 2 1

Library of Congress Cataloging-in-Publication Data

Reddy, S. Sethu K.
  The Cleveland Clinic guide to diabetes / S. Sethu Reddy.
    p. cm. — (Cleveland Clinic guide series)
  Includes index.
  ISBN 978-1-60714-073-3
  1. Diabetes—Popular works. I. Cleveland Clinic Foundation. II. Title.
III. Title: Diabetes.
  RC660.4.R43 2009
  616.4'62—dc22

2009013174

Kaplan Publishing books are available at special quantity discounts to use for sales promotions, employee premiums, or educational purposes. Please email our Special Sales Department to order or for more information at *kaplanpublishing@kaplan.com,* or write to Kaplan Publishing, 1 Liberty Plaza, 24th Floor, New York, NY 10006.

Contents

Introduction

Ben Dexter has just been diagnosed with diabetes at the age of fifty-six. He's upset, because he knows all too well about the disease, which affects approximately 30 million men and women in the United States.

Ben's father was diagnosed with diabetes in 1960 and died in 1989. According to Ben, "everyone else" on his father's side of the family developed diabetes and, until his generation, died from it. For years, many of Ben's relatives had warned him to take better care of himself in order to avoid becoming the next victim. A succession of doctors had dispensed the same advice. But he never changed his eating habits. Nor did he make an effort to exercise regularly.

So now, here Ben sits in his doctor's office, angry with himself for not doing more to sidestep the disease that has caused so much heartache for his family.

As a newly diagnosed person with diabetes, he's facing the very real prospects of eventually suffering one or more of the disease's many long-term complications: blindness, stroke, heart disease, pancreatic disease, kidney failure, nervous system damage, sexual dysfunction, and impaired circulation to the legs, possibly requiring amputation. Now he's scared.

Scared enough, hopefully, to take his condition seriously. The first thing that Ben needs to do is to become informed about diabetes and to sort out the truths from the myths. Then he needs to learn the many steps he can take to avoid those secondary maladies and live a long, healthy life. And he needs to understand, as we'll see, that he's not much different from many people in similar situations.

I'm going to presume that you're in a situation similar to Ben's: newly or recently diagnosed with diabetes. Or perhaps you've had diabetes for some time now and are looking to improve your control of the disease. Or maybe you're the concerned friend or relative of a patient. This book will answer all of your questions. It is full of up-to-date, essential information about diabetes, its complications, and the latest treatments.

Throughout, you will meet several people who talk candidly about their experiences with diabetes, from a Major League Baseball pitcher to a family where all the members have diabetes. You'll meet men, women, and children who have learned to manage the disease and take control of their lives. It's safe to say that in this day and age, *everyone* faces the possibility of developing diabetes or has at least one friend or relative with the disease (whether he or she knows it or not). So don't you think you should be prepared?

We hope that reading this book gives you hope. Even though diabetes is on the rise, our understanding of the disease is also increasing, along with research into new medicines and other therapies, and, most significantly, ways to prevent getting diabetes. You are the captain of your ship, and with the help of your family, friends, and your diabetes team, I'm sure that you'll be sailing through smooth waters.

Dr. S. Sethu Reddy, MD, MBA, FRCPC, FACP, MACE
Consultant physician and former chairman,
    Endocrinology, Diabetes, and Metabolism,
    Cleveland Clinic
U.S. scientific director for diabetes and obesity at
    Merck & Co., a global pharmaceutical company

Chapter 1

What Is Diabetes?

"What is diabetes?" is a surprisingly complicated question because the disease involves several organs and affects different people in different ways.

The short answer is that diabetes is a disease in which the body doesn't produce or can't properly use *insulin,* a *hormone* made by the *pancreas.* The body uses insulin to convert sugar, starches, and other food into the energy that powers us. We get sugar (*glucose*) from two sources: It's converted from the food we eat—specifically, from starches, or *carbohydrates*—and it's also manufactured in the liver and muscles. The pancreas releases insulin into the circulation, which helps glucose to enter various cells and be stored. If your body doesn't make enough insulin or if the insulin doesn't work the way it should, glucose can't get into your cells. It stays in your blood, causing your *blood glucose level* to rise too high, which is the condition we call diabetes.

If left untreated, diabetes can lead to heart disease and stroke as well as problems with the eyes (including blindness), kidneys, gums and teeth, sexual function, and nerves and blood circulation, which could eventually lead to foot or leg amputation.

Defining Diabetes

The way we determine whether or not a person has diabetes is by conducting a *fasting plasma glucose (FPG) test* or an *oral glucose tolerance test (OGTT)*. The fasting test works pretty much as you might imagine it would: A person's blood is drawn from a vein in the arm and tested for its glucose content after he has fasted for a certain number of hours. The oral test measures the blood glucose level following a fast *and* then again two hours after the patient has ingested a glucose-rich beverage.

Currently, a person is considered to have diabetes if the fasting sugar is 126 milligrams per deciliter (mg/dl) of blood or higher.

Why Is 126 Milligrams per Deciliter the Chosen Cutoff?

Until 1997, the number used to be 140 milligrams per deciliter. But based on some long-term observational data, it was determined that people with sugar levels above 126 mg/dl were more likely to develop eye complications, and so the diagnostic criteria was changed.

• • • *Fast Fact* • • •

In the metric system, 126 mg/dl is equal
to 7.0 millimoles per liter (mmol/l),
a nice, round number.

• • •

In the future, it's possible that the blood glucose definition of diabetes may have to be lowered further to account for the disease's effects on the heart or the peripheral blood vessels (the vessels outside of the heart and brain, particularly in the lower legs). That is, we may someday define diabetes as a fasting sugar greater than 105 or 110 mg/dl. Since the fasting sugar may not reflect what the sugars are like over the span of a whole day, there is some consideration of using the Hemoglobin A1C as a diagnostic test. Hemoglobin A1C reflects the average of the blood sugars over a two to three month period. You'll read more about this test later.

The current standard of 126 mg/dl defines diabetes based not on today's risk but on the future risk of developing a *complication* of the disease. Think of it this way: Certain medical conditions, like pregnancy, are discrete variables; a woman is either pregnant or not pregnant, and it's very easy to ascertain the pregnant state. But blood sugars are continuously variable, so definitively diagnosing diabetes depends on the likelihood of a certain outcome. There will always be a few people who develop complications even with only slightly elevated sugar levels, but we've chosen a level at which such complications are most likely to occur in most people.

Here's another comparison: You've probably wondered why the breathalyzer used by police to determine a person's blood alcohol level (BAL) is set to a certain number. I'm sure that somewhere there is data showing that a driver with a BAL of X or higher is more likely to have a car accident. So, for safety's sake, it is best for that person not to drive. In order words, the test doesn't measure inebriation per se; it establishes a standard blood alcohol level at which most people should not get behind the wheel.

Likewise for diabetes: A few people with fasting blood sugar levels below 126 mg/dl may develop eye complications in the future, just as many folks with very high blood sugars never experience complications. Your goal, regardless of your blood sugar level, is to reduce your chances of developing complications.

No matter how we define diabetes, we do know that as we get older, (1) our bodies become more resistant to insulin and (2) the pancreas secretes less insulin. This is why the prevalence of diabetes in young people may be 1 or 2 percent, but in the elderly it rises as high as 25 percent to 30 percent—that's 1 out of 4 people.

V.I.P. (The Vital Insulin-Making Pancreas)

The pancreas is a small organ that sits in the belly just behind and under your stomach. It has two main duties. One is to release substances called *enzymes* into the gut, to help you digest carbohydrates, fats, and proteins in the diet. Without these enzymes, we wouldn't be able to absorb the nutrients that we eat. The second function is to release many hormones into the bloodstream. The major hormones of interest are insulin, which comes from the organ's *beta cells*, and *glucagon*, from *alpha cells*. You already know that insulin helps the body store nutrients and lower blood sugar levels. Glucagon, on the other hand, raises blood sugar levels. To function properly, the pancreas must respond to our eating habits, especially when we eat. When we're not eating, the organ typically "rests."

How Can You Tell If Someone's Pancreas Is Working Adequately, Particularly with Respect to Insulin?

The next time you go to Thanksgiving dinner or some other social occasion, take a look around. If you see someone who has weighed 200 to 300 pounds for a long period of time and doesn't have diabetes, you can confidently assume that his pancreas has the ability to make sufficient insulin. Without adequate insulin action, a person will *lose* weight. However, if a person is losing weight and the sugars do not improve or even worsen, it's likely that the pancreas is beginning to fail and he or she will probably need insulin therapy to control his or her diabetes.

What's Happening in These Stages of Diabetes?

This is the final lap for the beta cells (the insulin manufacturing cells) and the pancreas. Perhaps 10 or 20 years ago, the person may have had what's called *insulin resistance,* where it takes more insulin to keep the blood sugar normal and to incorporate the nutrients into our tissues after eating. All this time, the pancreas has had to work harder, and eventually the beta cells give out. Once that happens, there isn't enough insulin to overcome the resistance, and blood sugars start rising.

Types of Diabetes

The major types of diabetes are *type 1* (so-called *juvenile-onset diabetes* or *insulin-dependent diabetes*) and *type 2* (*adult-onset diabetes* or *noninsulin-dependent diabetes*). All types of diabetes are related to either a lack of insulin levels or a lack of insulin effect.

What Is Type 1 Diabetes?

Type 1 diabetes is an *autoimmune disorder* in which the body's defense system misidentifies the pancreas as a foreign entity and attacks it, much like the way the body will reject a transplanted organ. People are usually diagnosed with type 1 diabetes under the age of 40, but we've come to recognize that many older men and women also develop the disease and require insulin therapy right from the beginning.

Type 1 diabetes is associated with several complications. Short-term health problems include *hyperglycemia* (high glucose levels in the blood), *hypoglycemia* (low blood sugar), and *ketoacidosis* (high blood levels of a chemical called *ketone*), while longer-term effects can include cardiovascular disease, blindness, nerve damage, and kidney damage. We'll discuss all of these, and others, in greater detail in later chapters.

It's still not clear what causes type 1 diabetes. We do know that it is highly genetic, yet it does not run in families like, say, brown eyes or flat feet. For example, in studies of identical twins, if one twin develops type 1 diabetes, the other twin has only a 50 percent chance of developing the disease. This is fascinating, since identical twins have identical genes! Therefore, it is thought that perhaps an environmental trigger—such as a virus or some toxin—tricks the immune system into destroying the pancreas.

A tremendous amount of research is under way trying to identify the early stages of diabetes and then to find ways to control the immune system to prevent destruction of the pancreas. It sounds like science fiction, but the future could bring a vaccine to prevent type 1 diabetes!

People with type 1 disease should pay special attention to eye care, foot care, skin care, heart health, and oral health in order to delay or prevent the onset of complications. There are things you can do to help, and there are also things you can avoid doing, too, like smoking and drinking excessive amounts of alcohol.

What Is Type 2 Diabetes?

Type 2 diabetes is more common than type 1, and it is more common in African-Americans, Latinos, Native Americans, and Asian-Americans/Pacific Islanders, as well as the aged. Most of the short- and long-term complications of type 1 mentioned above may also develop in people with type 2 diabetes. Traditionally, type 2 tends to be diagnosed later in life, but, increasingly, many young people who are obese and who have either a family history of diabetes or belong to the higher-risk ethnic groups are developing the disease earlier. It used to be that pediatricians would assume that every child with diabetes had type 1 and start them on insulin right away. But now that we know that some of these children actually have type 2 diabetes, pediatricians and family physicians are learning how to use pills and lifestyle measures to control these cases.

Type 2 diabetes is the result of insulin resistance as well as the pancreas's inability to supply the body's cells with enough of the hormone. As long as the beta cells can keep up with the insulin resistance, blood sugar levels can remain normal. But once the beta cells start failing, sugar levels rise.

It is thought that type 2 diabetes is a relatively modern disease, occurring in the past few thousand years. With increasing obesity and reduced physical activity occurring in populations with a genetic tendency toward diabetes, type 2 diabetes has become almost epidemic in some corners of the world. So it appears that both type 1 and type 2 diabetes are the result of interactions between our genetic background and our environment.

• • • *Fast Fact* • • •

Gestational diabetes: when diabetes develops during pregnancy but disappears after the birth; discussed in greater detail in chapter 6.

• • •

Back to the Future: Prediabetes

We should also mention *prediabetes.* This is a state in which a person may be at risk of developing diabetes. Many of these men and women may have what we call *dysmetabolic syndrome* or *metabolic syndrome:* a constellation of multiple risk factors for diabetes as well as for heart disease.

Individuals who fit this category typically carry a lot of fat in the middle of their bodies yet have relatively thin arms and legs. They may have fat accumulation in their livers, and they tend to exhibit altered levels of cholesterol and a form of fat called *triglycerides.* Typically, their "good" cholesterol (*high-density lipoprotein,* or *HDL,* cholesterol) levels tend to be low. Since a blood sugar level of 126 mg/dl or higher denotes diabetes, blood sugar levels between 100 and 126 indicate *impaired fasting glucose levels.* A person with blood sugar in this range may be deemed to have prediabetes. Some people will have a normal fasting sugar level but an abnormally high sugar level after taking a glucose load. This is called *impaired glucose tolerance (IGT).* A study by the federally funded National Institutes of Health (NIH) showed that lifestyle modification and about 150 minutes of exercise per week can significantly reduce the rate of diabetes, particularly among the elderly. Many other studies have also demonstrated that a healthy diet and regular physical activity have a tremendous impact on delaying the onset of diabetes.

Recent studies have found that medications such as metformin, pioglitazone, acarbose, ramipril, and rosiglitazone may prevent prediabetes from progressing to full diabetes, which would represent a great advance in medicine. Having said that, it should also be noted that intense debate exists about whether metabolic syndrome even exists. Still, it's useful for a physician to see this group of symptoms in one person. If insulin resistance is the root cause of many of the components of metabolic syndrome, then it makes sense to see if we can treat the insulin resistance and thus treat the whole metabolic syndrome.

Another debate raging in the scientific community is whether insulin resistance causes metabolic syndrome, or whether it's the increase in fat cells that then secrete a variety of hormones that can bring about metabolic syndrome. The problem is that it is extremely difficult to tease out the actual cause. One challenge in this area is that any intervention may exert an effect on both insulin resistance and fat cells. For example, exercise can reduce insulin resistance as well as the amount of fat.

This reminds me of the story of the 1854 cholera epidemic in London, England. The cause of the outbreak wasn't clear, but a physician named John Snow traced many of the cases to a particular water pump in the city. Snow's efforts greatly limited the spread of the disease. He didn't invent a miracle drug—he simply advised breaking the pump's handle so that Londoners couldn't drink its contaminated water. My point is that in medicine we don't always need to know the biochemical origin of a condition in order to arrive at a safe, effective treatment.

Diabetes Myths and Misconceptions

Unfortunately, many myths surround diabetes and its complications, thanks mainly to old wives' tales and bogus Internet sites. Even though abundant reliable information is readily available, it is sometimes difficult to separate the wheat from the chaff.

Let's take a look at some of the most common questions that patients ask about diabetes.

Can You Develop Diabetes by Eating Sugar? Does Having Diabetes Mean That You Must Avoid Simple Sugars or Sweets?

Eating lots of sugary foods does not cause diabetes. And a person with diabetes *can* eat sugar. It's the total number of calories that are important. (Too much sugar in your diet could cause cavities, though!) If you eat excessive calories of any kind, causing you to gain weight and become insulin resistant, then you may wind up with diabetes. Currently, the American Diabetes Association recommends that a healthy diet may include up to 15 percent of its calorie content from simple sugars, so long as the other 85 percent are derived from a healthy distribution of fats, proteins, and carbohydrates. Too often, people skip the sugar in their coffee but eat lots of fat and starchy foods. Don't get fooled into thinking that avoiding simple sugars is enough. Certainly, eating whole grains and vegetables which contain complex carbohydrates, along with lots of fiber, will be beneficial.

Everyone needs to watch his or her sugar intake. People who have or are predisposed to diabetes—that is, with a family history of it—need to be even more careful than most.

If I'm Overweight, Will I Get Diabetes?

Obesity does increase the chances of developing diabetes; the vast majority of folks with type 2 diabetes are obese, and 85 percent of people with diabetes are obese or overweight.

But not all obese people will develop diabetes; in fact, 80 percent of obese men and women do not have diabetes.

What this means is that other factors, combined with obesity, may give rise to the disease. In addition to increasing age, perhaps the most important risk factor is a family history. If you have a parent with diabetes and you happen to be overweight, the chance that you will develop diabetes is much higher than average. On the other hand, if you're overweight or obese but have no family history, you may be relatively protected against developing the disease.

Then there is the controversy regarding the active or fit overweight person. Someone who is overweight or obese but is physically active and exercises regularly may be doing him or herself a big favor in delaying the onset of diabetes. Obesity, family history, ethnic origin, diet, and physical activity all play a role.

Doesn't Diabetes Mostly Affect Older People?

Many of our parents or grandparents developed diabetes when they were in their fifties or sixties. But in the past 10 to 15 years, it has become increasingly evident that people in their thirties, twenties—and even in the teen years—are being diagnosed with type 2 diabetes. The implications of this are disastrous: If a person develop diabetes at age 15, then develops heart complications 10 or 15 years later, it's likely to shorten his life span. Furthermore, what if he has children who then have their own children? It's unlikely that these grandchildren will have any meaningful relationship with their grandfather. This will no doubt adversely affect both the cultural and social fabric of society. I call this the "metabolic tsunami." We've received a warning and now we need to do something about it.

Are Diabetes Medications Very Expensive?

The cost of medications is not usually a barrier to compliance, despite the fact that patients who fail to take their medications as directed frequently use this as an excuse. (In England, where drugs are distributed free, studies show a high rate of noncompliance nonetheless.)

If cost really is a problem, check with your physician for cheaper alternatives and with your insurance company about other ways to save on expenses. Many insurance companies

Noncompliance: Getting in the Way of Your Own Health

It's frustrating for physicians that some patients don't take their medications according to the doctor's orders. Even in a setting like a hospital or a nursing home, many people with diabetes will either forget to take their pill on schedule or refuse it entirely because they don't like the taste or fear the side effects.

You need to discuss the problem with your prescribing physician. Write down the exact reasons why you are forgetting or avoiding your medication. Maybe you need to carry a daily pill container for all of your medications wherever you go. Or you may need to have one set of pills in the bathroom and another set in the kitchen, and possibly another set in your briefcase or purse. (However, *do not* expose the pills to high temperatures, which may inactivate some of the medications.)

offer three- or four-month prescription plans where you can get a 90-day or 120-day supply for a greatly reduced price (like three months for the price of two). If you don't own your home and your income is low enough, you may qualify to get support directly from the drug manufacturer. Almost all of the major drug companies offer help to those who truly cannot afford their medications.

There has also been a trend of developing combination pills that may let you reduce your copay when you buy the medication. So instead of paying two copays for two different medications, you would pay one copay for a combination pill. Ask your physician if this might be appropriate for you.

Now That I Have Diabetes, What Can I Do to Stay Healthy?

Diabetes can be managed, like most things in life, but it takes effort. Develop good habits from the beginning, and the easier it will be to control the disease down the line. It's like buying life insurance: When you're young and healthy, the premiums are pretty low, but if you wait until you're elderly and ill to buy insurance, the cost will be exorbitant. So we can do a tremendous amount, but we need to get started earlier rather than later.

Stated bluntly, no one else is going to do this for you, so you have to take charge of your care and manage it from minute to minute, day to day, month to month, and year to year.

The good news is that medications are getting more convenient, as is self-monitoring your blood glucose levels. And thanks to new technology involving the Internet and the telephone, physicians, nurses, and dieticians are able to help manage their patients' condition. Slowly but surely, a virtual safety net is being built for everyone. Soon it will be like having your own private angel.

A Japanese proverb states that a thousand-mile journey begins with a few steps. One step at a time, and with some patience, you'll get to your destination safely.

Will Having Diabetes Shorten My Life?

People with diabetes can absolutely live long and healthy lives. Many new therapies are arriving on the market, and better systems to prevent diabetes complications are being developed. Those with diabetes can fare just as well as those without diabetes in respect to treatment of heart disease or obtaining kidney transplants. Years ago, many people with diabetes were excluded from kidney transplants and other major medical interventions because it was thought that that these procedures would be of no use and a waste of resources. However, we now know that people with diabetes can benefit as much or more so from these interventions.

So the reality of diabetes is that we have plenty of reasons to be optimistic about the future, and those who are diagnosed with diabetes today have a chance to write their own history, preferably with a favorable outcome.

Do All People with Diabetes Experience Complications Such as Kidney Failure, Blindness, and the Need for Amputation?

Certainly these severe effects can occur as a result of diabetes. However, only 30 percent of those with diabetes suffer end-stage kidney failure requiring dialysis or transplantation even after 30 years with the disease. We can tell if someone is developing kidney disease early enough so that we can intervene. By controlling your blood sugar, as well as your blood pressure and cholesterol levels, you may be able to protect your kidneys.

Also, it is extremely important to have your eyes checked annually. As we'll explain in a later chapter, your family physician or eye doctor should be able to see changes in your eyes before you have any symptoms. Here's more good news: If your doctor detects these indicators, he or she can initiate medical therapy or laser therapy to prevent vision loss. Your eye doctor can also monitor simpler problems like *cataracts,* which can be removed when the time is right. *Glaucoma* (increased fluid pressure in the eye) is more commonly found in those with diabetes compared to those without diabetes—but it can be controlled medically.

As for protecting your legs and feet, it's always important to inspect your feet daily by placing an unbreakable mirror on the floor. This will allow you to look easily at the tops and bottoms of your feet. When you check your feet, look for any breaks in the skin, unusual red or blue spots on the soles, or any changes in the arches or toenails. Compare one foot to the other to see if there is any difference. Whenever you step outside your bedroom, wear slippers or other footwear to protect your feet.

Remember: Just because you can't feel anything doesn't mean that everything is okay. People who have neuropathy and can't detect what they're stepping on feel unduly confident about their feet. Or their feet may look nice and pink, which makes them feel immune to foot problems.

It's always a shame when you learn that people who are losing their vision haven't seen an eye doctor for five or ten years, or you hear from an amputee that he walked around the beach or his backyard without any shoes and accidentally stepped on a nail or a child's toy but never noticed the injury. Many tragic situations begin with very innocent symptoms or events that slowly but surely get magnified. Then you learn that a mountain *can* be made out of a molehill—if you don't pay attention and care for yourself, that is.

If I Have Diabetes, Do I Need to Worry about Anything Other Than My Sugar Levels?

High blood sugar is just one symptom of diabetes; it is not strictly a sugar and insulin disorder. Diabetes is a complex metabolic illness that affects sugar, fat, and protein metabolism.

We now know that diabetes starts many years before high blood sugars develop. Many other changes precede the elevated blood sugar, including changes in your fat cells; changes in your blood vessels, which usually can be associated with increased clotting or elevated blood pressure; or an increased likelihood of responding poorly to certain medical stresses. Some would call diabetes a vascular disorder, with the high blood sugars a relatively late marker of those blood vessel problems. In diabetes, your blood vessels may be silently sustaining damage without your being aware of it until serious symptoms emerge.

Is It True That Women With Diabetes Cannot or Should Not Have Children?

Patients with diabetes can and do have children, although there are some risks involved. Women with poorly controlled diabetes at the time of conception may experience problems. Therefore, before she gets pregnant, she needs to get her sugars under proper control. We generally recommend that you complete your family as soon as possible if you have diabetes. A longer duration of diabetes or having complications of diabetes increases the risk of the pregnancy to the mother and the baby.

Will I Have to Take Insulin Shots If I'm Diagnosed with Diabetes?

Insulin therapy is not inevitable. Plus, there are many alternatives to having to inject yourself. Insulin isn't addictive and, in one sense, it's not even a drug; it is purely a replacement of our naturally occurring hormone insulin. Sometimes, as in the case of pregnancy, it's safer to be on insulin therapy. In some cases of infection, heart attack, or a major operation, people may need insulin temporarily to better control their sugars. Being on insulin for these circumstances doesn't mean that you'll be on insulin forever.

Many people remember an uncle or aunt who was placed on insulin after being admitted to the hospital for an infected foot, or with kidney failure or a heart attack. They then associate the initiation of insulin therapy with those complications. In truth, Uncle Joe or Aunt Sarah should have started taking insulin many years before. That way, their diabetes, cholesterol, and blood pressure could have been controlled to avoid the foot, kidney, and heart problems. Thus, although insulin therapy today can be more time consuming and demanding of a person's attention than managing the disease through diet, exercise, and medication, beginning insulin therapy earlier may help to delay or prevent complications.

Chapter 2

Symptoms of Diabetes

The challenge for all is that many men and women with diabetes think they don't have any symptoms. Often, a routine blood test may uncover the diabetes before symptoms occur.

The classic symptoms are increased thirst, increased urination, blurred vision, and fatigue. (See next page.) Too often, though, many of us think that we're just getting older, and so *of course* we're tired, and it's *normal* to put on more weight. We think it's natural for our vision to get blurry and to go to the bathroom more frequently. Then again, many older people don't experience the classic symptoms at all, possibly because elderly kidneys tolerate a higher level of sugar before producing more urine.

If your blood sugar becomes increasingly elevated, it can make your blood much more likely to clot, which can lead to strokes or heart attacks or problems with the peripheral circulation. High blood sugar can also affect our peripheral nerves, resulting in burning or tingling sensations, particularly in the feet, though they can occur anywhere in the body.

So What Exactly Are the Symptoms of Diabetes Onset?

The following symptoms can occur over a very long period of time. This is one reason why it can sometimes take five to seven years before diabetes is diagnosed. However, with type 1 diabetes, these symptoms may occur over the course of a few days—which is much more dramatic and more noticeable. Therefore, a person who develops type 1 diabetes is more likely to seek medical attention very soon and get diagnosed more quickly.

Frequent urination and increased thirst. The classic symptoms of diabetes are related to the elevation in blood sugar levels. In order for the kidneys to get rid of this excess sugar, they need to expel water and electrolytes as well. This necessitates making more urine, which leads to frequent urination or urination during the night. Of course, if you're passing more urine, you risk becoming dehydrated, so you feel thirsty and drink more water to keep up with the fluid losses. (Note: If you try to quench your thirst by drinking regular soda or fruit juice, which are full of sugar, this can elevate blood sugar levels even higher.) Frequent urination can also result in a loss of *electrolytes,* which can trigger other symptoms, such as muscle weakness and muscle cramps.

Blurred vision. The elevated blood sugar also can cause the lens in the eye to swell, resulting in blurry vision. Interestingly, a person may get used to the high sugars, and vision may return to normal. Then when we lower the sugar to normal, the vision may blur again, but only temporarily.

Fatigue and weight loss. Glucose is a form of energy. Since, in diabetes, the body cannot incorporate glucose into its cells (and energy cannot be stored in muscle and fat), a person with diabetes may feel fatigued and tired. When this inability to store energy becomes more serious, people actually lose weight.

Does Diabetes Affect My Heart?

It's becoming more and more evident that heart disease goes hand in hand with type 2 diabetes. Usually diabetes precedes the critical symptoms of heart disease by many years. However, the reverse pattern is also becoming more common, where patients who have had *angina* or other forms of heart disease or have undergone coronary artery bypass surgery are at a high risk of developing diabetes in the near future; so they should be checked for early warning signs on a periodic basis.

Are There Any Other Symptoms That I Should Be Aware Of?

Here are a few other symptoms that you may not know about, but should.

Frequent yeast infections for both women and men.
If you have recurrent yeast infections, you and your doctor should consider that you may have underlying diabetes. Yeast or fungal organisms thrive in a high blood sugar environment that may be moist. Thus, areas in the groin and under the breasts and arms are likely sites for recurrent fungal infections. Of course, you may have frequent yeast infections for other reasons—for example, sometimes women on birth control pills suffer from recurrent yeast infections—which is why it's important to see your doctor for a definitive diagnosis.

Delayed healing from superficial cuts and abrasions.
High blood sugar levels can impede wound repair and increase the tendency of wounds to become infected, which can also contribute to delayed healing.

Delayed gastric emptying. High blood sugar can slow down the ability of the stomach to push churned-up food to the small intestine, the next stop in the digestion process. This delay can bring about occasional nausea or a sensation of fullness even after eating a small meal. Sometimes, after many years of diabetes, damage to the nerves supplying the stomach can result in a type of paralysis of the stomach. As you can guess, this can play havoc with your diabetes control. For example, you can take your medication on time and eat on time, but if your meal is stranded in the stomach and doesn't get absorbed (the role of the intestines), your sugars can bounce up and down erratically.

Fatty liver. Sometimes high blood sugar levels indicate insulin deficiency, and this may be associated with elevated triglycerides (greater than 150 mg/dl). In this situation, the liver may make more triglycerides and also reduce the ability of fat cells to store them, resulting in a higher than normal concentration of triglycerides circulating in the blood. Chronically elevated triglyceride levels (greater than 1,000 or 1,500 mg/dl) can inflame the pancreas, a painful and potentially dangerous condition called *pancreatitis*.

It is quite common for the liver to overaccumulate fat, especially in type 2 diabetes. It is becoming increasingly recognized that a fatty liver is not just an innocent finding. It can eventually lead to *cirrhosis*—a life-threatening chronic

Red Flag

If you have three or more of these symptoms, make an appointment to visit your doctor right away. If you are at high risk, your doctor may decide to screen for diabetes anyway.

1. Frequent urination
2. Passing large amounts of urine
3. Increased thirst
4. Blurred vision
5. Fatigue or irritability
6. Sudden weight gain or weight loss
7. Frequent fungal infections
8. Delayed wound healing
9. Burning, pins and needles, or numbness in the extremities

Children and Diabetes

So far, we have no indication that diabetes slows a child's growth. Youngsters with diabetes typically reach their predicted adult height. But you need to watch for the other symptoms, especially with the incidence of childhood onset on the rise.

disease that scars healthy liver tissue until the organ no longer functions properly—and may also be associated with increased risks of heart disease and liver cancer. It is thought that if a patient's insulin resistance can be diminished, the fatty liver may improve.

Foot numbness. People with diabetes often experience sensations in their feet called paresthesias, which they tend to describe as a "pins and needles" feeling, prickling, or burning. This is due to nerve irritation. Any of these symptoms require prompt medical advice. It's paradoxical, but as nerve damage progresses, causing further numbness, patients frequently report less burning.

John's Story
John Canterbury has suffered through several medical problems, including diabetes. Like many people, before he was diagnosed with diabetes, he knew almost nothing about it. Another common problem comes through in his story: He doesn't get a lot of support at home in his efforts to combat the disease, which also seems to be the pattern with his

other ailments. And though he has tried hard to follow our suggestions, he still struggles a bit with some aspects of treatment—such as when and why to test his blood sugars. But he is trying, and as you'll see, he does have a pretty positive attitude.

I was diagnosed with diabetes when I was forty-three in 1992. I'm fifty-seven now. I think I know why it came down on me at that time. I was trying to get my disability because I had injured my knee—I had three knee surgeries—but despite my injuries, I didn't qualify because I was too young, they said. I couldn't work, I couldn't pay my bills. I was frustrated and depressed, so I sat at home eating oranges. I love oranges. I ate them by the dozens. I was also eating junk and drinking a lot of pop. I gained a lot of weight. I started off at, say, 230, 225, somewhere around there. But I went up to 300 pounds within a few months. I was just sitting home just gorging myself, and I started getting sick. I started shaking a lot; couldn't figure out what was wrong. I told my wife, "Baby, something's wrong with me."

She said, "Oh, nothing's wrong with you."

I said, "Oh, yes, there's something wrong with me. You know I don't like to go to the hospital, but call the hospital." And when she called and told them what was wrong with me, they told her to bring me in.

By the time we got there, I was just about out cold. I couldn't sit up, couldn't do nothing. My eyesight went; I couldn't see nothing, and I never wore glasses. I got there, and they took my blood and said, "His sugars are five hundred. He needs to be on insulin."

I asked Dr. Sethu Reddy, I think about the third time I saw him, "Is it possible for a person to go from the needle to the pills?" He said it's possible, but some people, once they get on the needle, that's it. I said, "No, that's not for me. I don't like going around carrying a needle and medicine. First thing people want to do is think you're a junkie. They start looking at you. No, I know I'm not going to do that." And I did the best that I could do. I exercised, I watched what I ate.

At first I couldn't figure out how I'd gotten sick, but I found out, you know, it's hereditary. My father has it. Right now he's in a wheelchair; he had a stroke when I was about twenty-four. He was putting in this lady's gas line, and he usually cuts the gas off when he puts the lines in, but this time he didn't cut it off, and as the gas blew past his nose, he went straight out. When he woke up, he was in a hospital and found out he had diabetes. Now me and him look just alike, and he always teases me. He says, "You come down with diabetes just like me. I know your blood is my blood. It all runs in the blood." Also, my grandmother on my mother's side died from diabetes long ago. So now I know.

I started exercising more, walking the dog or working out. I'd work out for at least twenty minutes, then I'd go sit down and chill out; I couldn't do too much because my knee would swell up on me. But I kept myself going, and after a while, I went from hypodermic needle to the pill Glucophage [metformin]. Oh, man, that is so much better than having to stick yourself.

I started eating NutraSweet instead of sugar. I watch my starches, all my starches. White bread, I don't eat, period. If it's not wheat bread, then I don't want it. I got hypertension too, and in 1993 the doctors told me that I'd had a "silent heart attack," and I didn't even know it. I don't eat much meat now. And I quit eating salt; I started eating salt substitutes. I've got reading glasses, so I take them with me to the store to read the labels.

I try not to eat any ice cream because once I start on some ice cream and it tastes good ... I used to go get a gallon of ice cream and eat half a gallon in one day just by myself. Now, peanuts, I love fresh peanuts in the shells. I look for the ones that say "no salt." They do have fat, so it depends on how many you eat. If you just eat a little bit, then it's not going to hurt you. And I eat fruits, but I don't eat a lot. A little bit here, a little bit there. I'm trying not to gain weight. I'm trying to keep my sugars and stuff down, so I watch everything I eat.

My wife and I, sometimes we eat different things. She tells me, "Your food is too bland. I don't like the way it tastes." So she'll cook herself something a little extra and put more seasoning in it. Sometimes she'll have meat with a lot of fat and everything, and I say, "Baby, you trying to kill yourself? You want to die before me? You going to leave this house to me? Because once you're dead, the house paid off, and I got nothing else to worry about."

She looks at me like I'm crazy, but I'm serious; her mother had diabetes, her sister has it now, her brother had it, and one of her nieces came down with diabetes when she was in the tenth grade. I keep telling my wife to get checked for diabetes, but she won't go. My stepson, he was here today and told me that his cholesterol seemed a little too high. He's thirty-one. I said, "Son, you're on the verge. Your grandmother had it, your auntie got it, your cousin got it." He looked like he was listening for the first time: Maybe I got across to him.

I hope I have.

Chapter 3

The Major Risk Factors

A re you at risk for developing diabetes? The main risk factors are genetic and environmental. Age is also a risk factor; as we get older, we have a higher chance of developing diabetes. In fact, more than 25 percent of people ages 65 and older have diabetes.

Genetic Risk Factors

Let's look at the genetic risk factors first. If one of your parents has or had type 2 diabetes, you stand about a 25 percent chance of developing diabetes during your adulthood. If both your parents have or had type 2 diabetes, you have about a 45 percent chance of developing it.

If you belong to a certain ethnic group, such as Hispanic, East Indian, African-American, Native American, or Asian, and you now live in a Westernized country, you have a higher chance of developing diabetes than people of European origin. It's interesting that even in these ethnic groups, within their native lands, people who live in an urban or modern setting have a higher chance of developing diabetes than those who live in a rural or traditional culture. The most striking example of this is the Pima Indians, who reside in the southwestern United States. Fifty percent of the adult Pima population has type 2 diabetes.

Diabetes is a relatively modern disease in these societies and was rarely heard of until 100 years ago. Although the people from these ethnic groups today are genetically similar to their ancestors from 1,000 years ago, it's clear that modernization and changing lifestyle patterns have demonstrated how susceptible these groups are to developing diabetes.

One theory about this is the so-called *thrifty genotype*. That is, over tens of thousands of years ago, our ancestors survived because they were better able to store energy, which helped them survive during lean months when food was scarce. This biological component enabled them to withstand feast-or-famine cycles. However, this ability to survive wild swings in nutrient availability may be unhealthy today, where we have plenty of access to food and nutrients and don't need to store energy for later. Thus, eating more fatty food and exercising less will lead to weight gain and possibly diabetes. This is an example of how a trait may be advantageous in one situation but a disadvantage in another. Being light and agile may help a baseball shortstop but not if he decides to moonlight as a sumo wrestler!

• • • *Fast Fact* • • •

Studies of twins provide another example that
illustrates how important your family history or
genetics might be. It has been shown that if
one identical twin develops type 2 diabetes, the
other twin has about a 95 percent chance of
developing diabetes as well.

• • •

So Is Obesity a Risk Factor?

Obesity is a major risk factor but, interestingly, from a
genetic point of view, if you're obese and have no family
history of diabetes, you have a low chance of developing
the disease. On the other hand, if you're obese and have a
family history of diabetes, you have a much higher chance
of developing the disease than an obese person without any
family history of diabetes.

Remember Ben from the introduction? While working
full-time as a comedian, Ben had kept himself in good condition, exercising regularly and eating a relatively healthy diet.
But as soon as he quit the stage and no longer needed to appear
before large groups of people, he also quit exercising and eating correctly, which meant giving in to his desire for sweets.
He gained weight rapidly, going from 135 to 190 pounds
in about two years—a dangerous situation for anyone but
especially someone who stands just five-foot-six. Such weight
gain is even more significant if there's a strong family history
of diabetes; as you know, Ben's father and nearly everyone else
on that side of the family had diabetes, with most of them
dying from complications of the disease.

If Ben did not have a family history of diabetes, his weight gain would still be of concern, but his chances of developing the disease would not be quite so high. It's the combination of genetics and obesity that really clinches it.

There's something else that Ben should be concerned about: He has two children, both young adults, who are also at risk for diabetes because of their family history. But, you may think, what do they have to be worried about; diabetes is an older person's disease, right? In fact, the fastest-growing segment of the population to be diagnosed with diabetes right now is adolescents. Given Ben's family history, the best course of action is for his children to start getting tested for diabetes now—and continuing to do so throughout their lives. They might also learn from their father's mistakes and live as if they had diabetes to prevent actually becoming so.

Environmental Risk Factors

Now let's look at some environmental risk factors. Factors such as weight gain, lack of exercise, and living in an urban, stressful environment can increase your risk of developing diabetes. (How is stress related to diabetes? Well, when we're stressed or anxious, we're likely to reach for a bag of fattening chips while parked in front of the TV instead of doing something that's good for us. Not everybody, of course, but enough of us.) In fact, when you combine both the genetic and environmental risk factors, there may be as many as 40 million Americans who could be classified as prediabetic and at risk of developing diabetes in the near future.

One of the more worrisome trends in recent years is the convergence of several risk factors involving younger age and a faster pace of life. We're seeing adolescents and young adults develop type 2 diabetes about 15 to 20 years sooner than their parents did. Our concern is that this new generation may be the first in history to have a shorter life span than the previous generation. This could have a major impact on family structure, social culture, and health care economics.

Perhaps the key environmental factor is the composition of our diet. It's been suggested that a high fat intake (especially *saturated fats, which* are solid at room temperature) may affect the way that insulin works, resulting in *insulin resistance* and thus a higher tendency to develop diabetes. (Conversely, a higher amount of fiber in the diet may slow the absorption of sugar and temper the rise in blood sugar after eating a carbohydrate-laden meal.) Although there is no data to suggest that dietary sugar causes diabetes, certainly taking in too many calories from one major source—whether it's carbohydrates, fats, or proteins—can lead you to put on weight gain and increase your chances of developing diabetes.

Other Risk Factors

Here are some other risk factors to consider:

Blood pressure and cholesterol. People who have high blood pressure or a cholesterol or triglyceride problem that's being managed through other medications are at higher risk of developing diabetes.

Smoking. Smoking has been identified as a risk factor for insulin resistance, which can lead to *hyperinsulinemia*—a condition where higher than normal amounts of insulin circulate in the blood. In addition, smokers with diabetes have a higher risk of heart disease. In one study of women aged 60 to 79 who smoked and developed type 2 diabetes, about 65 percent of them died from cardiovascular disease, which was attributed to the interaction of cigarette smoking and diabetes.

Alcohol. Drinking alcohol to excess may also lead to problems with the liver and with the way that insulin works, resulting in a higher chance of diabetes. Chronic excess of alchohol can cause inflammation of the pancreas. This can also lead to diabetes.

Conflicting medications. Another common risk factor is a medication that's being prescribed for another condition. For example, corticosteroids such as prednisone or dexamethasone, or high blood pressure medications like the diuretic hydrochlorothiazide, can increase the chances of high blood sugar. While these medications are necessary for medical treatment, your physician tries to find the lowest dose that will be effective for you.

Pregnancy and gestational diabetes. Some women develop diabetes during pregnancy, but after the baby is born, the disease disappears. This is known as gestational diabetes. It occurs in about 4 percent of all pregnancies but is more prevalent among African-Americans, Hispanic/

Latin-Americans, and Native Americans. It's also more common among obese women and women with a family history of diabetes.

Pregnancy can stress the pancreas. Approximately half-way through a pregnancy, a woman becomes more insulin resistant; therefore, her insulin secretion may be inadequate, resulting in diabetes. (Normally, the blood sugars are lower during the first three months of pregnancy, so the criteria for diagnosing diabetes are little more stringent than in non-pregnant women.) The placenta provides most of the nutrition for the baby and also makes a number of hormones that can aggravate insulin. It can also metabolize insulin quickly. Thus, usually after delivery, these risk factors disappear, and the mother's sugar status reverts to normal. However, all is not *quite* normal. Women who develop gestational diabetes have a 5 percent chance of developing type 2 diabetes in the five to ten years following the delivery. And once a woman has had gestational diabetes, the chance that it will return in future pregnancies increases.

The Bottom Line

Look at yourself in the mirror and carefully jot down any genetic risk factors and environmental risk factors that you think may affect you. We certainly can't change our family history, so there's no point worrying about that. Focus on the environmental risk factors that you are exposing your body to and try to minimize these risks. If we can help the 30 million at-risk people in the U.S. avoid diabetes, then we'll be doing society a huge favor. On the other hand, if these 30 million people develop diabetes, it will be a huge setback for gains in our medical system.

Chapter 4

Short-Term Complications of Diabetes

The goal of diabetes treatment is to prevent the variety of complications that people with diabetes are vulnerable to. Over time, diabetes can injure the heart, kidneys, eyes, blood vessels, and nerves, and you may not even know damage is taking place.

Strictly controlling your blood sugar level is the key to minimizing your risk of complications. However, even the very best control may not be able to eliminate all complications, and the risks increase over time. Therefore, it's important to be vigilant.

In the next two chapters, we'll discuss some of the complications that may arise from diabetes, starting with short-term effects.

Hypoglycemia

Keeping your blood sugars low is probably the best thing that you can do to control diabetes. But if the sugar falls too low, you may experience shaking, sweating, intense hunger, and anxiety.

Maintaining a healthy blood glucose level is very much like walking along the edge of a cliff. Staying balanced is the key. If you're in good control of your diet and your sugars remain very close to normal, you have a higher chance of the sugars occasionally slipping below normal. So I always tell my patients that if they are taking hypo-glycemic drugs and are in good control, they may have two or three very mild low blood sugar episodes per week.

On the other hand, if you rarely experience a low blood sugar reaction, your diabetes control probably isn't very good. Because if you have high blood sugar—let's say 200 mg/dl—then even if it drops by 50 points to 150, you still won't fall into the hypoglycemic zone. However if your sugars are averaging between 100 and 120—a healthy level—you may occasionally experience low blood sugar reactions when you overexercise or wait too long between meals.

In men and women without diabetes, we generally consider them to be hypoglycemic if their blood glucose level tests below 50 mg/dl. However, we generally advise people with diabetes to treat sugars when their levels drop below 70. We tend to be more cautious with those who are on medical therapy. With some individuals, if the sugar falls rapidly— for example, from 250 to 100—that rate of sugar drop may result in some symptoms of low blood sugar, even though technically the person is not hypoglycemic.

What Happens When Blood Sugar Drops Too Low?

It's important to remember that our body is equipped with two lines of defense against hypoglycemia. The first comes from two hormones from our nervous system: *adrenaline* and *acetylcholine*. When the sugar level in the circulation drops below normal, these hormones are released. This can result in shaking, increased sweating, rapid heartbeat, and hunger. If you raise your blood sugar level right away, the symptoms will subside. However, if you do not notice these symptoms or ignore them, the sugar could fall further. Secondly, with sugars falling below normal, the pancreas releases glucagons, which "tells" the liver to release sugar into the bloodstream. The brain depends on the blood to bring it glucose for energy. If it doesn't receive enough, a person can find it difficult to focus and experience slight personality changes, a blank or vacant stare, confusion, and/or disorientation. In extreme hypoglycemia, sufferers can begin to seizure or even fall into a coma. This is why it's very important to be aware of the early symptoms of low blood sugar, to avoid these subsequent effects on the brain.

Which Diabetes Medications Are Associated with Low Blood Sugars?

The medications taken by people with noninsulin-dependent diabetes are intended to keep blood sugar levels from climbing too high. Sometimes, though, these drugs do their jobs a little too well, driving the level down too low. However, the risk of hypoglycemia is minimal with medications such as acarbose, which blocks sugar absorption from the small bowel; metformin; and *thiazolidinediones* (TZDs for short) such as roglitazone or pioiglitazone. A new class of agents, known as the *gliptins,* also are associated with a low risk of low blood sugar, as is a new injectable drug called a GLP-1 analog. These medications are less likely to cause low blood sugars on their own.

However, any drug that stimulates insulin release from the pancreas, independent of the glucose level, can bring about low blood sugar levels. For example, the oldest class of oral agents for diabetes, *sulfonylureas* (SFU), stimulates insulin secretion and may at times cause low blood sugar. People at high risk for this reaction are the elderly, those with a tendency to skip meals, and those who have had diabetes for a long time. Kidney failure patients who take SFU medications may be particularly prone to hypoglycemia.

Of course, even insulin itself, in excessive amounts, can cause low blood sugar. But how do you define an excessive dose? Everyone is different and needs different levels and amounts of insulin to control his or her diabetes. Thus, one person may be well controlled on 20 units of insulin a day, while another person might need 150 units. Simply put, if you keep experiencing hypoglycemic episodes on a certain dose of insulin, then you and your doctor can probably conclude that *for you* the dose is excessive.

Hormones and Blood Sugar

A low blood sugar level prompts the pancreas to secrete the anti-insulin hormone glucagon, which causes sugar to be released by the liver. Other hormones that are stimulated by low blood sugar include *cortisol* from the adrenal glands atop your kidneys and *growth hormone* from the pituitary gland located at the base of the brain. These hormones have much-delayed effects, but they are very important in maintaining glucose stores in the liver and muscle.

If someone experiences a hypoglycemic episode for a very short duration and is able to recover by himself, we call this a mild hypoglycemic episode. But if he needs someone else's assistance to recover, it is considered a severe episode. Severe hypoglycemia typically occurs in people who have lost the adrenaline-and-glucagon response to low blood sugars. The quartet of hormones referred to above—adrenaline, glucagon, cortisol, and growth hormone—are considered counter-regulatory hormones. A patient with type 2 diabetes rarely loses this ability, but someone with type 1 may lose the counter-regulatory response after 10 or 15 years of diabetes.

You can prevent hypoglycemic episodes by being more consistent with your diet, physical activity, and medication usage. Whenever these variables are out of sync, you could experience a low blood sugar reaction. A note of caution about exercise, however: Many people occasionally exercise intensively, and when they check their sugar immediately afterward, it appears fine. What they don't realize is that their muscles are still active metabolically and can continue to take up glucose from the blood; thus, they may experience hypoglycemia two or three hours *after* exercising.

Then there's the "let the punishment fit the crime" method of treatment. Too often, when someone's sugar drops, he becomes very anxious and irritable—almost panicky—and tends to overreact to a low blood sugar by overeating. Typically, you should treat a hypoglycemic reaction with a small snack that includes about 15 grams of carbohydrates. It can be in liquid form, such as a half glass of orange juice or a half can of soda. Then wait 10 to 15 minutes for the symptoms to improve. If you don't feel any better, try snacking again.

Sometimes people continue to eat even after they're feeling better. What they don't realize is that the very first snack they ate 15 minutes earlier did the trick. If you manage low blood sugar episodes in this manner, you'll end up with very *high* blood sugars after the initial low blood sugar. The way to go, then, is to snack modestly and wait 15 minutes. This will provide smoother control with less weight gain, despite the occasional hypoglycemic episodes. It's also better to snack while you're having symptoms; don't think that you can put off eating. Some people will tell themselves that since lunch is in a half hour or so, they can hang on. But sometimes the sugar will drop further, worsening the situation. If you have sufficient time, a protein snack and simple sugars would be ideal, since protein tends to maintain the sugar elevation for a longer period of time.

• • • *Fast Fact* • • •

There's a new twist in this: Some snack foods are made from cornstarch, which can delay glucose absorption and thus may be ideal for preventing hypoglycemia in the middle of the night.

• • •

> ## Red Flag
>
> If you have severe low blood sugar today, chances are high that in the next 48 hours, you may experience another severe low blood sugar episode.

Glucagon Injections

For those taking insulin and having severe low blood sugar reactions, we always try to train patients' spouses or significant others in how to recognize a hypoglycemic episode and how to administer an injection of glucagon to reverse the symptoms. Typically, 1 milligram of glucagon can be given just beneath the skin (*subcutaneously*) or into a muscle (*intramuscularly*). The hormone, which comes in powdered form in a vial and has a long shelf life, needs to be mixed at the time of injection. It usually improves the person's condition enough that he can drink or eat something.

Ketoacidosis

Ketoacidosis, typically seen in type 1 diabetes, is a condition of absolute insulin deficiency. In situations involving extreme stress, glucagon and other counter-regulatory hormones increase. This causes a high glucagon-to-insulin ratio, which forces the liver to burn fat for energy and generates ketones—an acidic substance produced when the body uses fat instead of sugar for energy. By this time, the cells are starving for glucose. In this particular state, blood sugar levels rise, ketones rise, and the blood's *pH* (the measure of a solution's acidity or alkalinity) drops. A low pH indicates that the blood contains too much acid. Patients in ketoacidosis breathe rapidly; what they're doing is trying to blow off the acid through the lungs in the form of carbon dioxide.

Ketoacidosis is typically a medical emergency. (Before the discovery of insulin, it was the leading cause of death from type 1 diabetes.) Normally, a person suffering from ketoacidosis is admitted to a hospital's intensive care unit. We control it by administering saline and insulin into a vein (*intravenously*). The usual goal is to bring down the blood sugar to about 200 mg/dl level, after which we become more conservative with respect to the rate of sugar drop. Then the patient is observed very carefully until he or she is transferred to a regular hospital floor.

Hyperglycemic Hyperosmolar Nonketotic Coma (HHNC)

This is a medical emergency in which a person with type 2 diabetes has enough insulin to prevent the fatty acids from being burned but not enough insulin to regulate glucose in the circulation. The blood sugar soars dramatically—up to 1,000 mg/dl or higher. (For a point of comparison, consider that even in poorly controlled diabetes, the level typically swings between 100 and 200 mg/dl. Occasionally, blood sugar might go higher than 300 mg/dl, perhaps from an extra slice of cheesecake at dinner or drinking too much fruit juice while watching a baseball game.)

One feature of HHNC is severe dehydration, which is more difficult to correct than you might think. A catch-22 develops: As the sugar level rises, the patient urinates more frequently and in large amounts. He can't drink enough to offset the fluid loss, so he becomes even more dehydrated, and the sugar concentration in the blood continues to climb. It is estimated that patients who present with hyperglycemic hyperosmolar nonketotic state are close to three gallons of water in the negative balance.

In addition to severe dehydration, the blood may become more concentrated and thick, causing it to flow more slowly. And when blood slows down, it has a tendency to clot, so you're more likely to get blood clots in your legs and elsewhere. If the circulation to the brain is impaired, the patient may experience strokelike symptoms and altered mental status, and may lapse into a coma.

The treatment for hyperosmolar ketonic coma is surprisingly simple: intravenous fluids, fluids, and more fluids to correct the severe dehydration. The results can be miraculous. As the blood sugar lowers, the patient becomes stronger, more alert, and the symptoms reverse completely.

Important: If, while measuring your blood glucose at home, you receive a reading of 300 mg/dl or higher, and it continues to rise, seek medical attention immediately. Don't wait until the level reaches 500 mg/dl or higher. In truth, most glucose monitors on the market register high values only when the sugar exceeds the range of the machine. Seeking medical guidance when the sugar hits the 300 to 400 mg/dl range could spare you the dangerous effects of extremely high blood sugars. In this case, an ounce of prevention is definitely worth a pound of cure.

What Happens After a Hyperglycemic Hyperosmolar Nonketotic Episode?

Sometimes hospitalized patient will need insulin to control their blood sugar temporarily, but once they've been adequately rehydrated, it's possible that they could resume oral medications or take a slightly different combination of oral medications. In some cases, a nondiabetes-related factor may have triggered the rise in blood sugar, such as pneumonia or some other infection. So having an episode like this doesn't necessarily mean that you'll need insulin for life.

• • • **Fast Fact** • • •

Hyperglycemic hyperosmolar nonketotic syndrome is more likely to occur in the elderly or those who live alone—in other words, those who don't tend to seek medical attention at an early stage.

• • •

Infections

Infections are a cause of concern to those with diabetes, because high blood sugars impair the immune system's ability to fight bacteria, viruses, and fungal infections. The immune system is made up of circulating white cells that kill foreign agents and produce *antibodies,* whose job it is to recognize the intruders if they should return to the scene of the crime. Normally, when a bacterium or a virus enters the body, a white cell called a *macrophage* (Greek for "big mouth") engulfs it and destroys it internally. But an elevated blood glucose level limits the macrophages' effectiveness. Bacteria escape their clutches and are allowed to multiply, resulting in an infection.

High sugar levels also offer an ideal environment for fungal growth. You've probably noticed this with food left for too long, say, in a bachelor's refrigerator. When the sugars are elevated, we're more prone to yeast infections, especially women, and fungal infections in the nails or other parts of the body. This is an important infection because it often develops before a person has been diagnosed with diabetes. So if you get repeated infections, your doctor should screen for diabetes.

People with diabetes are prone to other infections such as tuberculosis, which was eradicated in the late 20th century but is now making a comeback, since vaccinating against the disease is no longer a public health policy. I'm particularly concerned about tuberculosis in people who come to America from countries such as China and India, where they may have been exposed to TB and have a residual hidden infection that can run rampant once their blood sugars become elevated.

Foot infections are also a real danger. Along with the high blood sugars, if you have reduced blood supply to the foot and the skin is thinner or dry and cracked, your defenses against bacteria are greatly diminished. All it takes is one little cut that goes unrecognized and becomes infected. Infection can then progress deep into the skin and tissue below; it can even reach the bone. We call this infection of the bone *osteomyelitis*. When this happens, you have to take antibiotics intravenously for three months or more.

If the infection can't be eradicated, then we may have to resort to surgically removing part of the foot. Infection is usually the reason that people with diabetes must undergo foot or leg amputations. (We'll discuss the importance of foot care in chapter 6.)

Other infections you should be aware of are pneumonia and the flu. Among diabetes experts, the general feeling is that people with diabetes are no more likely to contract the flu than those without diabetes, but they tend to have more severe symptoms as well as suffer complications. Thankfully, most of us have access to flu shots. Unless you're allergic to eggs or some other component of the vaccine, it's highly recommended that you get vaccinated in the fall, before flu season. I also advise patients to get inoculated against the pneumococcus bacterium, the culprit behind a major form of pneumonia. This vaccine can help protect you for five or six years.

No vaccination can guarantee that you won't get the flu or pneumonia, but it will greatly reduce your chances of developing the flu of the year as well as the most common type of bacterial pneumonia.

Bladder infections and kidney infections are also more common with diabetes. So if you experience a burning sensation when passing urine or a change in urine color, call your physician. If you develop high fevers and back pain along with these urinary symptoms, you may have a kidney infection, which is a medical emergency that calls for immediate treatment.

Chapter 5

Long-Term Complications of Diabetes

W hen your doctor breaks the news that you have diabetes, it is normal to think, "That's not possible." Then you may wonder, "If only I had joined the Y a few years back, maybe things would be different." Finally, you come to accept the diagnosis and search for solutions to preserve your health.

You understand—and your family and friends need to understand—that diabetes can't be put away and taken out periodically. It's a lifelong acquaintance that stays with you, wherever you go and whatever you do. You will need to maintain your energy level and self-manage your diabetes to prevent the long-term complications.

We classify chronic, long-term complications of diabetes into two groups:

- *Microvascular* (affecting small blood vessels)—complications of the eyes, kidneys, and nervous system.

- *Macrovascular* (affecting large blood vessels)—heart disease, stroke, and poor circulation in the legs.

Microvascular Complications

Vision Problems

Diabetes is the leading cause of adult blindness in North America. It's also one of the complications that we can detect directly when we examine someone's eyes.

In the back of your eye is the *retina,* which can be compared to the film in a camera. The retina is made up of specialized nerve cells that detect light and receive nourishment from blood vessels. In diabetes, these blood vessels, especially the smaller ones, are fragile and may suffer small hemorrhages—bleeds—in the back of the eye. Several years later, this may lead to *proliferative retinopathy:* the growth of new blood vessels in the back of the eye.

Unfortunately, these new vessels are even more fragile and much more likely to rupture. While minor hemorrhages are common and relatively harmless, excessive bleeding near the retina can greatly impair a person's vision. For example, since 95 percent of our most precise and color vision is located in one tiny spot on the retina called the *macula,* bleeding near the macula will significantly affect our ability to see and may even lead to blindness. The changes caused by all these new blood vessels and excessive bleeding can result in *fibrosis,* or scarring of the retina. When the retina becomes scarred, it can lift itself off of the back of the eye, very much like a poorly laid carpet lifting off the floor. *Retinal detachment,* as this is known, brings about further vision loss. However, expert retina surgeons can try to repair this.

Fortunately, we can prevent blindness from proliferative retinopathy by zapping the area of new blood vessel growth with a laser beam. We can safely laser the rest of the retina and protect the macula, thus preserving vision.

Glaucoma (glaw-*co*-ma) is a condition where the pressure in the eyeball is abnormally high. It's akin to having an overinflated tire. Excessive pressure in the eye can damage the retina and could eventually lead to blindness. It's not usually painful, and that's why you should get your eye pressures checked at each formal eye exams.

Cataracts, a disorder of the lens, mainly affects older people. In diabetes, however, the lens is even more prone to clouding up over many years. How do you know whether you should consider cataract surgery to remove the damaged lens? It depends not so much on how cloudy the lens is but on how this affects your vision. If you see halos around streetlights and traffic lights at night or have trouble seeing at night in general, it may be time. I remember when cataract surgery required a one-week hospital stay, and patients were left with these striking eyeglasses and odd-looking eyes. Now this is a one-day procedure, and the surgeon can usually replace the cloudy lenses with prescription lenses. No one can tell whether you had cataract surgery or not. Many can even do without their old eyeglasses!

An Eye Examination Schedule

If you have type 2 diabetes, you may have had the disease for five years or more without realizing it, so it's recommended that you have your eyes examined by a qualified provider at the time of diagnosis and then yearly. If you have type 1 diabetes, we usually know when the disease actually started. Since retinopathy is relatively rare, early on, men and women with type 1 diabetes should see their eye specialist within the first year. Follow-up visits can be scheduled according to the doctor's recommendation.

People with diabetes may also be more prone to *sties,* inflamed swellings in the *sebaceous glands* of the eyelids. This, in turn, can lead to *conjunctivitis,* an inflammation in the white part of the eye. So it is essential to practice good eye hygiene when you wash your face every morning.

Though all of these eye complications can be serious, often a patient will still see reasonably well while all these changes are occurring in the back of his or her eye. This is why it's so important to have regular examinations with an expert ophthalmologist or optometrist—these professionals will spot hemorrhages and other changes in your eye long before you may notice any vision problems.

Good eye care includes watching your blood pressure. As with most complications of diabetes, prevention is the key. In addition to regular eye exams, you want to maintain healthy blood pressure, which for most folks is no higher than 130 mmHg (millimeters of mercury) over 80 mmHg.

Red Flag

It's critical not to dismiss vision issues as just "eye problems." Quite often, eye problems go hand in hand with kidney problems. If I see a patient who has diabetic retinopathy, I always suspect that there might be some underlying kidney damage as well.

Persistently elevated blood pressure, or *hypertension,* can inflict further damage on the blood vessels in your eyes—not to mention increase your risk of suffering a heart attack or stroke.

If you are diagnosed with hypertension, treating it aggressively will protect your eyes

from the ravages of diabetes, as will adequate blood sugar control. We can't ensure that you'll never experience eye problems, since even people with fairly good blood sugars and good blood pressure can develop retinopathy. It's a bit like driving home after having had too many drinks at a holiday party—chances are that you'll get home safely, but the chances are also higher that you'll have an accident. On the other hand, if you're sober and drive home, you reduce your chances of a car accident, but your risk never truly goes down to zero.

Kidney Disease

Having diabetes doesn't guarantee that you will ultimately develop kidney disease. In fact, only 30 percent of men and women who have lived with diabetes for 30 years will have end-stage kidney problems. That said, diabetes is still the leading cause of end-stage kidney disease in North America.

Decades ago, when someone with diabetes developed renal failure, it was almost the end of the road. *Hemodialysis* (see below), carried out in a hospital or dialysis center, could be hard on patients' lives. In 1976, however, *peritoneal dialysis* was perfected. This method, which patients perform themselves—at home, at work, or wherever they happen to be—likewise removes wastes from the blood.

Hemodialysis and Peritoneal Dialysis

Hemodialysis is the process of taking blood from one of your veins, running it through a filtration unit (artificial kidney), and then returning the purified blood back to you. Since our blood contains not only waste material but millions of cells as well as vital enzymes and nutrients, it is important that the "good stuff" is kept. Hemodialysis is usually performed three times a week, with each treatment session typically taking three to five hours. You will be surprised to know that folks can travel internationally and even go on cruises and get dialyzed there.

Peritoneal dialysis takes advantage of a membrane in our bellies. Simply put, the patient infuses about a gallon of sterile sugar cleansing solution into a tube that's been surgically implanted in the abdomen and lets it sit there for four to six hours while going about her business. During that time, some of the waste chemicals from the blood cross the *peritoneal membrane* into the sugar solution. After several hours, the used fluid is drained out, and a fresh bag of solution is put into the belly. This must be repeated three or four times a day.

Kidney Transplantation Surgery

In the past, doctors avoided performing kidney transplants on their diabetic patients because most physicians believed the operation was too great a risk. The medications used to prevent kidney rejection after transplant surgery also tended to exacerbate the diabetes and thus lead to poor outcomes. Thankfully, better antirejection medications are now available. In addition, better dialysis regimens and improved preventive care are available in case kidney failure occurs.

With kidney disease, the question is: Can we see the train coming before it hits us? The short answer is yes. The kidneys are efficient, constantly filtering all the components of blood. Proteins, too, get filtered. It's been found that diabetics with early kidney disease may have more protein in the urine than normal. One protein in particular, called *albumin,* is our main focus of interest. Significant amounts of albumin in the urine, even though the kidney appears to be functioning well, is a red flag to physicians that they need to take more caution with kidney care and kidney protection. We can detect this problem early with a *microalbuminuria urine test* to identify traces of albumin in the urine.

Blood sugar control, whether you have type 1 or type 2 diabetes, can reduce the onset of kidney complications by up to 35 percent. Lowering your blood pressure will also protect the kidneys and slow end-stage kidney disease. Blood pressure medications such as *angiotensin converting enzyme (ACE) inhibitors* and *angiotensin II receptor blockers (ARBs)* appear to protect kidney function even further by having an additional effect on the kidneys.

Many people think that as long as they're passing urine, their kidneys must be working properly. This is a great misunderstanding. It's possible to have very good urine formation but still have damage being done to the kidneys, so it's important that people with diabetes get their urine checked once a year at their physician's office and pay attention to their blood pressure, cholesterol, and blood sugar levels. Remember, with diabetes the complications are very intertwined. Vigilance is critical to long-term health.

Certain people with type 1 diabetes with end-stage kidney disease may be good candidates for not only a kidney transplant but also a pancreas transplant. Combined pancreas-kidney transplantations are being performed with increasing frequency. This makes sense because the transplant patient will be taking antirejection drugs to protect the kidney, and these same drugs may help protect against rejection of the pancreas. It may also improve kidney function and possibly cure the diabetes, at which point the person would no longer need insulin therapy.

Improved blood sugar control will also increase the longevity of the transplanted kidney. One year of dialysis can cost up to $60,000, so protecting the kidneys for longer and longer periods of time will not only save the patient's life, but also preserve the health care budget for years to come.

Nervous System Disorders (Diabetic Neuropathy)

Diabetic neuropathy (nerve damage) is a very common complication. Up to 25 percent of people with type 2 diabetes may have mild neuropathy even at the time of diagnosis. The symptoms of neuropathy are widely varied, and since neurons exist throughout the body, symptoms can occur in almost every organ. The most common type is *sensory-motor neuropathy,* which involves the nerves that supply our skin and muscles, and the classic symptom is numbness in the feet, starting in the toes and gradually progressing upward to the ankle, knee, and beyond. This is the so-called "glove-and-stocking" distribution of neuropathy. In addition, when the nerves that supply muscles are damaged, the muscles will tend to waste away, resulting in muscle weakness.

Special facial nerves control our eye muscles, allowing us to move our eyes from left to right and up and down, and the muscles that facilitate smiling, laughing, and chewing. Diabetes can suddenly affect these nerves, so that a person may wake up unable to move an eye or experience weakness of the facial muscles. Damage to another nerve can cause changes in hearing. These types of neuropathies are unusual in that not only can they occur very quickly, but they can completely disappear two to three months after their onset. Nevertheless, the symptoms can be frightening.

Gastroparesis. Nerves that supply our heart, stomach, intestines, sweat glands, and many organs that are beyond our conscious control make up the *autonomic nervous system.* The autonomic nervous system consists of two competing systems: the *sympathetic system* and the *parasympathetic system.* For example, I can instruct my hand to move, because those nerves are under voluntary control; I can't order my heart to beat faster or tell my stomach to digest slower, because those are involuntary actions—they happen on their own.

Let's look at these systems one organ at a time. When the parasympathetic system in the heart gets damaged, the heart begins pumping faster, even when the person is resting. The system also plays a role in maintaining our blood pressure when we stand up. If it wasn't working properly, every time we stood, our blood would heed the laws of gravity and pool in our feet. Our brain wouldn't receive any blood, and we'd faint. People with longstanding diabetes may find that their blood pressure drops too much too quickly when standing up.

The autonomic nervous system also regulates our stomach and intestines. Often, an early sign of diabetes is constipation. When my son was about two years old, he realized that there was a neural connection between food intake and bowel movements. He quickly figured out that when he ate, within an hour or two, he'd have to go to the bathroom. This is called the *gastrocolic reflex.* In longstanding diabetes, this reflex may be reduced, and thus the movement of the colon is reduced—which we experience as constipation.

Beyond constipation, the stomach itself slows down. Normally, your stomach muscles contract and release, contract and release, churning up food and moving it along toward the small intestine. The name for this wavelike motion is *peristalsis.* Nerve damage from diabetes causes *gastroparesis*—literally, paralysis of the stomach. The soupy undigested food gets hung up in the J-shaped organ, producing discomfort and, occasionally, vomiting. The bigger problem for people with diabetes is that gastroparesis plays havoc with their metabolism, and, subsequently, complicates blood sugar control. You may time your insulin injections perfectly and eat right on time, but because the food now takes longer to be absorbed, your blood sugar spikes two hours after you injected yourself. When blood sugars swing this way, we call it "brittle diabetes."

We treat gastroparesis by advising patients to avoid high-fat foods and to eat a softer, perhaps even puréed diet, to allow swifter transit of food to the intestines for digestion. Sometimes we'll move insulin therapy to after meals, rather than before, so that the hormone injection can better match the rate of glucose being absorbed from meals. Your doctor may decide to try some medications to help your stomach and bowel to move things along. Some may even consider a type of "pacemaker" therapy to stimulate your bowel movement.

Peripheral neuropathy. For *peripheral neuropathy,* a painful condition accompanied by a burning sensation, we would suggest acetaminophen (brand names: Tylenol, among others) for analgesic relief or antidepressants, which seem to have an effect on this painful neuropathy. Duloxetine (Cymbalta), a cousin of the *selective serotonin reuptake inhibitor* fluoxetine (Prozac), except that it acts on two neurotransmitters instead of one, appears to help painful diabetic neuropathy. Other antidepressants have also been used, as have agents related to antiseizure medications. Both may provide benefits. There have been some reports, primarily from Europe, that alpha lipoic acid or sphingolipids, two nutritional additives, may also alleviate some of the nerve symptoms. An interesting treatment is capsaicin ointment or cream. Capsaicin is the active ingredient in green chili peppers. It burns initially but then has a numbing effect. Thus, it may help with painful neuropathy in the feet. Some have suggested mixing crushed green chili power with a cold cream cosmetic for a homemade capsaicin cream. Be careful with the amount of the active ingredient. Many of these agents may not be officially approved by the U.S. Food and Drug Administration (FDA) for this indication. You should check with your physician as to what is most appropriate for you.

Macrovascular Complications

Vascular Disease (Heart Attack, Stroke)

Diabetes is a major risk factor for the development of vascular disease because it can affect blood vessels in the brain, heart, and in the extremities. For people with diabetes *and* high blood pressure, this is like smoking next to a dynamite storage shed. Compelling studies conducted in San Antonio, Texas, show that at the time diabetes was diagnosed in the participants, the major blood vessels in their necks had already become narrower. From this we can imagine that similar narrowing is going on in the blood vessels in the brain and the heart, too.

Blood vessels are complex hollow tube-shaped organs made up of muscle cells and an inner lining of *endothelial* cells that acts as a barrier between the muscle tissue and the circulating blood. High blood sugar, as seen in diabetes, may affect the vessels as well as components of the blood, such as *platelets*. These are the cells that initiate clotting if you cut yourself and bleed. That's good. When a diabetic's blood glucose level spirals out of control, the platelets become "sticky" and more likely to clump together as they travel the

Red Flag

1. Women are normally less likely to get heart disease than men, especially before they enter menopause. Diabetes undermines this protection factor; therefore, women with diabetes have the same chance of developing heart disease as men without diabetes. After menopause, diabetes increases the risk of heart disease even more.

2. The targets for blood pressure control are even lower for people with diabetes than for those without the disease. Instead of 140/90 mm Hg as a target, we would like the blood pressure to be less than 130/80 mm Hg.

3. The same holds true for cholesterol levels. In fact, we treat people with diabetes as if they've had heart disease. Typically, if someone has a normal cholesterol level yet suffers from heart disease, then that level of cholesterol is too high for him or her. It doesn't matter that for thousands of other people, that cholesterol level may be okay. One approach for tackling the problem of a blood vessel disease in a person with diabetes is to try to lower the cholesterol, no matter what the level. Currently, the mantra is "the lower, the better."

   My personal opinion is that if you have heart disease, you should try to lower your cholesterol even if it has been in the normal range.

circulatory system. A clot lodged in one of the arteries to the heart triggers a heart attack; if the artery leads to the brain, a stroke. And here's yet another circulatory hazard: Hyperglycemia increases the number of *free oxygen radicals,* which play a part in hardening artery walls.

High concentrations of cholesterol or triglycerides in the blood, meanwhile, can also aggravate the endothelial and muscle cells. The vessels' inner walls hoard more and more fatty substances, which accumulate and constrict the opening—further setting the stage for heart attack or stroke.

• • • *Fast Fact* • • •

A diet rich in fiber (oats, flax, psyllium) in your diet can help lower your cholesterol. Also, some margarine-type spreads have plant sterols, which can also help reduce your cholesterol levels.

• • •

Does Diabetes Increase the Likelihood of My Having a Stroke?

Strokes are sometimes nicknamed "brain attacks." Diabetes certainly increases the chances of blood vessel disease in the brain. If the sugars are high at the time of a stroke, there's a chance that the stroke will be more damaging and recovery will be slower and less complete.

The very simple, cheap intervention is to take a baby aspirin (ASA) daily to prevent heart attacks and strokes. If you can't tolerate ASA, other non-ASA alternatives are available. Currently, some of this evidence is unclear. Some recent studies from Japan and Scotland have not shown a benefit from ASA. You should check with your physician as to the latest consensus.

Of course, taking care of your blood pressure and cholesterol levels will also help in preventing a stroke.

Other Long-Term Complications

In addition to microvascular and macrovascular complications, diabetes may affect other parts of your body or areas of your health. Some of these seemingly minor complications have more serious implications: For example, people with diabetes are more likely to have the gum disease *gingivitis,* a known risk factor for heart disease.

Gingivitis is also thought to be associated with insulin resistance. So it's very important for people with diabetes to take good preventative care of their teeth and gums, not only to save their teeth but, hopefully, their heart as well. So make sure that the dentist is part of your diabetes team!

Stomach Ailments

You've read about the nerve damage in the stomach and bowels, which can be associated with nausea, full feeling in the stomach, and constipation. However, paradoxically, diabetes can also cause diarrhea. There could be many causes for the diarrhea and if it is a persistent problem, you should see your doctor and may need to see a stomach specialist (gastro-enterologist). Treatments depend on what's causing the diarrhea. Changes in diet, anti-diarrhea medications and sometimes treating the underlying severe constipation may be necessary.

Bladder, too

Diabetes is not selective about which nerves it affects. As you can guess, our bladder automatically contracts when it's full.

If the bladder can't sense how full it is, it will keep stretching. So, one can develop an enlarged bladder and the urine can overflow and lead to incontinence. If you're a male, you will want to make sure that your prostate is healthy since an enlarged prostate can cause urinary flow problems.

What Does Insulin Have to Do with Sleep Apnea?

Up to one-third of diabetes patients may have a form of *sleep apnea,* which shouldn't be thought of as merely a benign disorder. Sleep apnea, long associated with a higher risk of heart disease and sudden death, has recently been associated with insulin resistance as well. Correcting the sleep apnea will enable you to sleep better and feel much more rested when awake. This will improve your energy during the day for increased activity and exercise, which may result in some weight loss, better insulin sensitivity, and improved blood sugar levels.

It's estimated that close to one-third of Americans overall suffer from sleep disturbance. When you combine this statistic with the high prevalence of diabetes, it's no wonder that many people with diabetes have sleep disturbances—which can make diabetes control difficult.

Will Diabetes Affect My Sex Life?

The combination of neuropathy and poor circulation from diabetes can result in *erectile dysfunction;* in fact, it is the leading cause of ED. It used to be that little could be done for this, but now we have several medications that improve a man's ability to maintain erections. Besides the obvious benefit, all the publicity (and frequent jokes on late-night talk shows) surrounding these drugs has helped doctors to broach the subject of sexual function (and dysfunction) more easily with their patients. That's a positive development, because sometimes ED may be a sign of a more sinister ailment, such as coronary heart disease.

Three oral medications—sildenafil (Viagra), tadalafil (Cialis), and vardenafil (Levitra)—are about equally effective at combating male dysfunction. They work by enhancing the effect of nitric oxide, a gas that figures prominently in the hydraulics, so to speak, necessary for an erection. Side effects of these drugs include visual changes; they should not be combined with certain heart medications, so check with your doctor about whether they could benefit you.

Although much of the focus has been on male sexual function, it's clear that diabetes may impact on female sexual function as well, particularly after menopause or in women who have *peripheral vascular disease.* Some early studies found no negative effect sexually in women with type 1 diabetes, but a significant effect on women with type 2. One theory is that women who develop diabetes during childhood experience minimal sexual problems later in life because they've grown into adulthood with diabetes as part of their self-identify; whereas if a middle-aged woman suddenly learns that she has type 2 diabetes, it may alter her body image and sense of self, which may have a secondary impact on her sexual function. This concept has been suggested for many disorders. For example, informing patients that they have high blood pressure can affect their self-perception. Remember though, psychology aside, the negative effect of diabetes on blood flow can adversely affect female sexual function.

Vasodilating medications such as Viagra have not demonstrated any benefit for women.

For postmenopausal patients, *estrogen replacement therapy* (ERT) may be beneficial to restoring normal sexual function. However, you need to check with your physician about all of the risks and benefits of hormone replacement therapy for you as an individual. You will hear lots of conflicting news stories on estrogen therapy. See what applies to *you*.

I've Been Feeling a Little Depressed More Often Than Usual; Can Diabetes Affect My Moods, Too?

Often overlooked amid all the discussion of blood vessel problems is depression, which has been noted in up to 20 percent of patients with type 2 diabetes. One reason why it may go unrecognized is that several symptoms of depression, such as fatigue, sleep disturbance, and a general loss of interest in life can be features of uncontrolled diabetes, too. Moreover, we've learned recently that depression is associated with insulin resistance and may also contribute to patients' difficulty following a lifestyle improvement program.

Depression may be directly related to your diabetes, or it may be a normal reaction to having been diagnosed with a serious illness that necessitates changes in your lifestyle. It can be difficult for some people to cope with such changes emotionally. Regardless of the cause, depression is a serious illness in and of itself that should be treated with care. If you have noticed any changes in your mood—including those noted above, as well as disinterest in socializing or unexplained feelings of despair—and/or if there is any family history of depression, let your physician know.

When I was a naive medical student, I imagined that if everything was okay in one's life, there was no need to be depressed. I quickly learned, though, that depression is often associated with biochemical changes in the brain and that you can't simply talk your way out of depression. It's important to be aware of these changes and to seek medical and spiritual attention.

Prevention Is Protection

The complications of diabetes are serious, to be sure. Fortunately, there's much we can do to prevent diabetes-related diseases of the eyes, kidneys, and nervous system. The mainstay of prevention, for these and all other complications, is managing your blood sugar. That is something only you can control.

Don't compare your situation with that of previous generations of diabetes patients. The technology and knowledge available have changed dramatically. For instance, we can detect symptoms earlier than ever before and thus initiate treatment sooner. I always tell my patients, "You can rewrite the history of diabetes for yourself. Don't be concerned about what happened twenty years ago."

If you have diabetes, remember this short list of things you can do to protect yourself:

1. Get your eyes checked once a year.

2. Get your urine checked once a year, along with a blood test for kidney function.

Tip

You may want to schedule some of these checkups close to the time of your birthday. It's an easy way to remember. It's a shame that we take better care of our cars than our bodies!

---

3. Keep your blood pressure below 130/80 mm Hg.

4. Keep your *hemoglobin A1C* at 6.5 percent or lower if it is practical and safe.

5. Keep your bad (LDL) cholesterol below 100 mg/dl and your good (HDL) cholesterol at 55 mg/dl or higher for women, and 45 mg/dl or higher for men. Try to cut down on animal protein in your diet and increase vegetarian sources.

6. If you do have early kidney impairment, see a *nephrologist* (kidney specialist) soon.

Jason's Story

Major league pitcher Jason Johnson, at six-foot-six and about 220 pounds, looks pretty healthy. He probably doesn't fit most people's image of a person with diabetes. Signed by the Pittsburgh Pirates in 1992, he hit the majors in 1997 and has played for the Baltimore Orioles, Detroit Tigers, Tampa Bay Rays, Los Angeles Dodgers, Boston Red Sox, and both teams from Ohio, the Cincinnati Reds and the Cleveland Indians. He is now in the Yankees organization. He used to duck into the clubhouse between innings to check his blood glucose level and then either gulp down a sports drink if his numbers were low or give himself an insulin shot if the numbers were high. Then, a few years ago, he got an insulin pump, and, as they say in sports, he's been pumped up ever since.

I was diagnosed with diabetes when I was eleven years old. I was born in '73, so that was '84. My mother was working at the time as a respiratory therapist, so she knew the signs and symptoms of the disease. I'd been having frequent urination at night; getting up six, seven times a night. And I'd drink water all night long—get up and drink, then dehydrate, and so on. And I was losing a lot of weight, too; I lost about twenty-five pounds. I was a pretty decent-sized guy, and I definitely thinned out. We lived in northern Kentucky, and Mom brought me to the Children's Hospital Medical Center in Cincinnati for tests. Sure enough, it turned out to be diabetes.

I really didn't have any idea of what diabetes involved. I mean, I was worried, but I knew I had to get shots and eat at certain times, and that was kind of tough on me at that age. I was in the hospital for a week and a half and was on two insulin shots a day at the time. After I got out, I had to go back every three and a half weeks or so to do a checkup to make sure things were going okay.

My mother gave me the shots at first, and when I got used to it—about a month into my treatment— I started doing it myself. I definitely felt the difference when I started getting the insulin. I mean, I was always real tired and just kind of didn't want to get up; just wanted to lay down all the time, you know. But you get a lot more energy when you go on insulin, and I wanted to go out and play with my buddies and stuff like that, and do sports again.

Doctors pretty much wrote everything out for me: This is what you want to eat in between meals, this is what you want to eat at meals, stuff like that. They were pretty strict about what they wanted me to eat in the beginning. Slowly, I changed my diet into what I wanted to eat and counted everything myself. I didn't really count calories; it was more like I had three bread exchanges, that kind of thing. I went by exchanges at the time: one fruit exchange, one milk, stuff like that. It was a little different back then.

When I first started testing my blood, I wasn't really excited about that part, you know; I didn't like it. I tested three times a day, and that was only at the major meals. And the testing device was massive, the size of a pretty big case—it was like a bookcase-type thing. It took about a minute and a half to two minutes to read it. I'd take readings before meals and then pretty much adjust my insulin accordingly: a little more if my blood sugar reading was high, a little less if it was a little low. So I took the insulin, and I had to eat at certain times every day or I'd have low blood sugars.

I came out of high school and went right into baseball. My parents told me, "Don't let diabetes stop you from doing anything. If you want to be a baseball player, we're going to stand behind you one hundred percent." That's what I wanted to do, so they stood behind me through my whole high school career.

When I signed with the Pittsburgh Pirates, I pretty much told the team doctors what kind of schedule I was going to have once I got there: early morning workouts, working out every day, and stuff like that. I met with a dietician and endocrinologist and got an idea of what they thought would be the best thing for me.

I eventually got an insulin pump five years ago, while I was with the Baltimore Orioles. I was introduced to somebody from the Medtronic company. With the pump, I'm more like a normal person; I can eat whenever I want to, get up whenever I want to. I used to have to get up at eight o'clock every morning, no matter what, and take a shot, but now if I want to sleep in, I can. If I want to eat a candy bar, I can; I dial it in on the insulin pump and eat a candy bar. It's a big difference.

I have to adjust the pump; it's trial and error. I count the carbs and just flip it in on the meals I had, dial in how much insulin to cover meals and things like that. It took about a month, and I got it to handle pretty much every type of food there is.

I actually check my blood more often now than before I had the pump—not because I really have to but because I'm more concerned with getting my blood sugars under better control to avoid any complications later in life. I do it six, seven times a day just to be more careful.

The needle goes in with a tiny infusion set, like a little tube around it, and I do it in my stomach or my hip. I can pull the needle out and the tube stays in. It doesn't get in the way of playing baseball; I really don't have any idea that it's there.

Having diabetes hasn't caused any problems in my career. I think that some teams might be a little reluctant to sign me because they may not understand what diabetes is and how to deal with it. But once I get on a team and talk to them and show them what it does and how it affects me, they're pretty understanding. I've been playing for eight years in the Major Leagues, so teams have seen what I've done, and they're pretty positive about it. The Indians have been really good about it.

I've pretty much used baseball as a platform to spread the word about diabetes. During the baseball season, I talk to groups. I'm going to meet with our public relations department soon about stuff I'm going to do this year with diabetes kids, talking to them and doing certain things to help them out. It's something I enjoy doing.

Every place I've played, I've met with organizations that deal with diabetes and helped them out in any way that I can. I know it can be inspiring to some kid who's been diagnosed with it and thinks he has to quit playing baseball or whatever sport he's into. I get letters all the time from young kids and their parents that say "You really made a difference in my child's life. They felt they weren't going to be able to do anything, and now they are." Stories like that keep me going.

Chapter 6

Controlling Your Diabetes

People who have been diagnosed with diabetes may feel like they've been dealt a bad hand. But in the game of poker, as in life, not everyone is dealt a great set of cards. Take a look at the really good poker players: Even when they're handed a poor combination of cards, they have certain strategies and techniques of minimizing the loss to fall back on; then they move on to the next game and, they hope, a better chance.

Jason continues to inspire us. He recently had a diagnosis of a rare type of eye tumor and after treatment, he continues to pitch professionally.

When we plan a family vacation, we look at our budget, the time of the year, tune up the minivan, and make sure the pet is taken care of and the mail is put on hold. That's just a small list. In managing your diabetes, you also need to plan ahead, taking the necessary precautions.

To manage your diabetes, you need to have a road map in mind, with a full and rich life as the theme of your journey. It's also important to know what the targets are. Too often, a person will see his or her physician again and again without really knowing what to aim for. This wastes a lot of time and will usually end up with the neither patient nor the physician happy.

Only if you, your friends and family, and your health care team are on the same page can you succeed. For example, what would happen if you knew what you should eat, but your spouse didn't think dietary compliance was important?

Self-Management

Trying to achieve the best blood sugar control is like driving 200 miles per hour in a NASCAR race. It's exhilarating, but there will be an occasional flat tire or a bump, and sometimes a major accident. However, if we stay on top of our game with a well-tuned car and all of the safety precautions, we can minimize these mishaps. Remember, you are in control.

In medicine, the current buzzwords are *self-management* and *patient empowerment*. The old word was *compliance*, meaning that we obeyed someone else's orders. Self-management and empowerment, on the other hand, mean that you've thought about your actions—both their impact and rationale—and are now self-motivated to carry out those actions. The "orders," therefore, are no longer from doctors or nurses or dieticians, they're yours. So when it comes to taking your medications, dining out, exercising, and your medical appointments, think about why, how, when, and what you're doing (or not doing). In this scenario, you are the CEO of your diabetes.

Jenny Asher has a thing or two to say about self-management. When Jenny was still married, four out of six people in her immediate family had diabetes: her husband and three of their four children. Of the children, the youngest was diagnosed first, and, as Jenny tells it, because he was so young, she "became diabetic for him." She worked hard to manage three kids' diabetes. It was difficult, but it paid off, and they're managing themselves now.

Jenny's Story

I have four children. When Mary was about eight and Michael was five, and Jim and Liz (the twins) were two, Jim got very thin, and he was always thirsty. One day while I was out shopping, my then husband tested Jim's blood with his own meter. The kids' father is diabetic, and his father was diabetic. My then husband had been type 1 since he was five. And his father got it when he was about twenty-seven.

Jim's sugar was so high it didn't register, so we rushed him down to emergency. They gave him insulin right away. He was prescribed several shots a day—with each meal and then in between if he was running high, or in the evenings, and he also had a bedtime shot. It was really hard because he was so young. I tried not to make a whole lot out of it, and there was a lot of busyness around us anyway. He was one of four kids, and I guess that helped. And with his father being diabetic, it wasn't abnormal to see those kinds of things happen. He didn't like it, but I didn't have to chase him out of the closets or anything. He was very brave.

Still, he was getting several shots and taking several blood tests a day. I became diabetic for him. He was two; I had to know everything he ate and how much, because I was in charge of his insulin.

For birthday parties and things like that, I'd call ahead and talk to the parents about what they were serving the kids, or else I'd have him eat before the party. But I'd let him have cake and ice cream—because if I didn't, I know that if somebody did that to me, I'd find a way to eat in the closet, and that's no way to live. I didn't ever want him to feel bad about his diabetes. I didn't allow him to go overboard, so we regulated his insulin and made sure his sugar didn't rise too high. It's either that or else he's going to eat it another time, and his sugar will be out of whack, so we trained him not to overeat, and that wasn't a problem. Although the doctor probably would not be happy.

When Jim was nine, his father had been on the insulin pump for about a year, and he talked the doctor into putting Jim on an insulin pump. I couldn't find anyone else anywhere else in the country who had a child on an insulin pump. I was so worried because I was the one in control of what he ate and how much insulin and all that. But he was very mature; he gave himself a shot when he was five. We were sleeping, and one morning he came and said he gave himself a shot because he was going to have breakfast. We didn't know what to do; do you praise him or what? Because we didn't know how much insulin he got, we had to watch him. But he took the first step toward managing his own illness, and that was pretty cool.

He quickly learned what to eat and what not to eat. He counted carbohydrates and knew how much a piece of bread was or how much half a piece of bread was, and then he could estimate things from there. But we had charts; there was a carbohydrate chart on the closet door, so he could refer to it when he ate breakfast. We read labels—he read labels—we counted carbs and estimated how much he was going to eat, and then he had a sliding scale for his insulin. The doctor taught him how many units for how many carbs he was going to eat, and he did that.

When Jim was in elementary school, I had a good relationship with the school nurse. I taught in the same school district. The nurse had to call me in my class- room because if Jim was low, the doctor needed my okay to adjust his insulin. And you can't just sign a paper, because the amount of medication given changes. Actu- ally, they would just hand the phone to Jim so I could talk right to him. He'd tell me what his number was and I'd say, "What did you eat last?" and "Well, what do you think? Do you think you need to take a couple glucose tabs or a couple of units of regular?" And he would tell me, and I'd agree or adjust it, but I'd try to let him think he was doing it. I had to, because I had to trust him to help me figure out what he needed when I couldn't be there.

By hearing him on the phone, I could tell where he was, too, and then I'd always talk to the nurse again; tell her that he sounds okay or he needs something right now, and I'd give them the okay. They made a special chart for Jim because there were no children at the time getting shots at school. I don't know what other diabetic kids were doing; maybe they didn't have other diabetics in our school system. Now it's not unusual for a school to have three or four insulin-dependent kids at any given time.

Jim did continue to get better control. The insulin pump gives him a minute amount of constant insulin, and you can program it to give larger increments and even put it in immediately when you need it. Having all of that gave Jim a lot of freedom. He still has the pump. He's learned to move it around. He used to put it just right on his tummy, and now he moves it around. He has more options now.

Then when Michael was fourteen, and in the ninth grade and playing sports, he came to me while he was training for wrestling, and he started complaining about his eyes. "Mom, I can't see; everything is all blurry." I told him we'd get his eyes checked.

He'd just come off of football season, where he won a couple awards. I wouldn't have suspected diabetes. But then at the same time, now that I think about it, he was real big on orange juice and grapefruit juice, and he drank them by the jug. And then he started complaining about peeing a lot. So we tested him here, everybody was here, and we just lost it. It was really a bad time.

The sugar was off the charts, so we took him down to emergency. He worked with the diabetes for about two years before he went on the pump. He got put on the pump when he was about sixteen, and that has made it a lot easier for him. He's twenty-two now. Mike and Jim have the same kind of pump, so it's nice that they can talk about the programming, how it works, supplies, and that sort of thing.

Mary was in college, and one spring my husband went down to visit her. She complained about having to pee a lot, and he, right away, said, "That's one of the symptoms, and we should check you out." And they did, and she was diabetic.

Jim's twin sister, Liz, hasn't been tested. It's her choice if she wants to, but she seems healthy, and there are no indications.

All of them seem to be managing diabetes on their own now. They like to be private about it, and I don't pry too much, but I do ask them, "So how's your sugar been?" I simply ask them as a way to bring it to the forefront, as a way of saying, "This is so important; don't give up on it, don't quit testing your blood, don't quit watching your sugar." Because I can't tell them what to eat or what to do. I never could. You just have to show them the right way.

Are you ready to take charge? Here are a few things to keep in mind.

Hemoglobin A1C

One of the first questions I ask new patients is whether they've ever had a test for three-month average glucose control, or hemoglobin A1C, and if they have, what the number is. Only a few know about the test, and even fewer know the results of their test. But you must know your targets; otherwise you'll never know how well you're handling diabetes.

The second important point is that most of the time, the targets are second-class. For example, it seems that everyone lets the diabetes go as long as the sugar levels are less than 200 mg/dl. But the diagnosis of diabetes is made when the fasting blood sugar is more than 126. In the course of managing diabetes, you can see that this doesn't make any sense. Like that old expression, "close" counts only in horseshoes and hand grenades. In basketball, you score points when the ball goes into the basket; you don't get any points for *almost* dunking it through the hoop.

The goal for each person with diabetes is to safely get his or her blood sugars into the normal range. The normal hemoglobin A1C range for people who don't have diabetes is 4 percent to 6 percent. To get to a count of 6.5 percent or lower, you need to have a fasting blood sugar close to 100 mg/dl or better, and a blood sugar two hours after eating, close to 140 mg/dl. These are difficult goals. If you can safely only get to 7.0% or 7.4% A1C, that's ok. Remember that any goal has to be *your* goal and not necessarily someone else's.

A landmark 2008 study, "Translating the A1C Assay into Estimated Average Glucose Values," published in *Diabetes Care,* a journal for health care practitioners, suggested that a certain level of A1C can imply an approximate average blood glucose level. We can call this an *estimated Average Glucose (eAG)*.

Table 1. A1C and eAG

Hemoglobin A1C %	eAG (estimated Average Glucose) mg/dl
6	126
6.5	140
7	154
7.5	169
8.0	183
8.5	197
9.0	212
9.5	226
10	240

Caution: An average does not reveal the highs and lows of sugar values. It's like your daughter's report card. Her average for the semester may be 85 percent, but if her math grade was

A1C Levels and You

For some groups of people, such as African-Americans, children, and pregnant women, the A1C may not equal the same eAG as in nonpregnant Caucasian adults. Check with your doctor or diabetes educator as to how reliable the test is for you.

> **Tip**
>
> For more information about *estimated Average Glucose,* including an online eAG calculator, visit the American Diabetes Association website at *http://professional.diabetes. org/glucosecalculator.aspx.*

100 percent, and she got only a 70 percent in English, she would know that she needs to try bringing up her English grade.

So it's important that you check your daily blood sugars as frequently as you and your physician think necessary to complement the information that A1C and eAG provide. Using eAG and your daily blood sugar checks can help improve your overall diabetes management.

Blood Glucose Testing

Blood tests provide your physician with a lot of important information, and it can give you information, too. Your doctor will discuss with you how often you should check your blood sugar. If you're testing, say, four times a day—before breakfast, lunch, dinner and then at bedtime—that helps us identify at what times of the day your blood sugar levels are running high or low. Journaling additional information about what you're eating and your activities throughout the day can further help us pinpoint what might be causing these spikes and drops; it could be from food or other things that can be adjusted, like your medication.

Some Practical Tips for Monitoring Your Glucose Levels

The Monitors

When glucose monitors were introduced in the 1980s, the devices cost more than $300. It took upward of several minutes to get a reading, which depended on the degree of color change on a glucose-sensing strip. Today's monitors are very affordable and are packed with extra features. They can be linked to your cell phone or even to your personal digital assistant. They can also report the sugar level within a few seconds.

The Lancets

The amount of blood needed to perform the test has come down more than tenfold; thus the needle prick itself has become less invasive. Almost every patient uses a spring-loaded triggering device to prick the skin with the lancet. The advantages are that the needle prick is very fast and only as deep as needed to obtain the blood sample. When patients try to do this manually, they will often hesitate and prick the skin too shallow or too deep.

Make sure that you adjust the lancet device for the right depth of skin penetration. Most devices have dials to adjust for the thickness of the skin. For example, if you work with your hands a lot, you're likely to have thicker skin.

Theoretically, there are 20 places in all to obtain blood. You have 10 fingers—use them all, so that no digit gets favored. Also, instead of inserting the lancet into the middle of the fingertips, aim slightly off-center, on either side. Not only does this double your number of potential targets, it's less painful.

(Continued on next page)

So-called noninvasive monitors are still in development. Don't be fooled by advertisements touting monitors that supposedly don't require sampling from your fingers. Strictly speaking, the claims are correct, but you have to prick your arm or your palm.

The Strips

The test strips have advanced tremendously. Many years ago, you had to differentiate among various shades of grayish blue and, later, various shades of blue green. Now the strips are high-tech and send a variable electrical signal to the monitor, depending on the sugar concentration.

Since the strips are manufactured in batches at different times, you may have to calibrate the strips for your monitor, depending on the batch. It's like baking cookies on different days: even though you follow the same recipe, the batches may turn out slightly differently. Calibration means that the monitor adjusts itself depending on the batch of strips. Check your monitor and your strips to see if you have to calibrate manually or automatically. You may also have a test solution containing sugar; placing a drop on the strip can also be used to test the monitor.

A good method to test your monitor is to bring it with you to your doctor's office. If the nurse can compare the office monitor with your monitor, using the same drop of blood, you will get an idea of how your monitor is functioning. Remember, though, that you shouldn't expect the two numbers to be identical. If the office monitor reports 120 and yours reports 130, that's close enough to be considered reliable. But if the office monitor reports 120 and yours reports 90, the difference is too great.

Your blood test tells you about the effects of what you just ate or what you ate three or four hours ago. This is invaluable information, but only if you act upon it. Too often, I see patients' diaries packed with blood sugar results showing that every evening they become hypoglycemic, or that day after day they have high blood sugars around breakfast time. But they make no changes in response to the tests, which defeats the whole purpose. If you're experiencing consistent abnormalities in your monitoring, you should think about modifying your behavior, medication, dosage, or timing. If you're not sure how to evaluate your results or how to make adjustments, ask your health care provider. Ideally, you'll be sharing your results with your physician periodically, although at the beginning of treatment, it's a good idea to do so more frequently so that you can both get an early handle on your particular situation.

People often ask about urine tests. Urine testing for sugar has gone the way of the dinosaur. Today a small sample of blood from a finger prick can be analyzed in five seconds or so. We're also rapidly moving toward glucose sensors, surgically placed under the skin for three to five days, that will automatically check the glucose level every five minutes.

I Really Hate Testing My Blood; Is It Okay to Do Them a Little More Randomly Instead of So Many Times a Day?

Blood testing can be uncomfortable, and a busy schedule may make it difficult for you to stick to a routine of testing and recording your blood sugar levels. However, without "sugarcoating" it, the fact is that you have a choice: the inconvenience and mild discomfort of regular testing, or serious complications such as blindness, kidney or heart failure, numbness in your extremities, and more. People with diabetes can lead relatively normal lives, but you must manage your disease consistently.

Some people are fooled into complacency because they take random readings that don't seem to reveal any negative patterns. But the fact that your random readings seem unremarkable doesn't necessarily indicate that everything is fine. It's important to see what your levels are every day, at different times of the day—that is, the same times every day—so we get the overall picture, which can tell us a lot.

You might be able to reduce the frequency of testing if your lifestyle is consistent and your diabetes is stable, with predictable glucose levels.

• • • *Fast Fact* • • •

The first "glucose monitor" was invented in India thousands of years ago. A physician would spill a sample of the patient's urine onto the ground, then see how fast ants would crawl toward the urine spot. Thus, he would be able to judge how high the patient's sugars were!

• • •

Urine Tests

Urine tests are still the mainstay of checking for ketones. As you learned in chapter 4, when insulin levels are extremely low in people with type 1 diabetes, the body turns to fat for sources of energy and produces ketones. In most circumstances, this usually indicates that the person's blood sugars are extremely high. We normally advise patients that if their sugars are running above 250 or 300 mg/dl consistently, they should check their urine for ketones. Today some blood glucose monitors also check for ketones in the blood.

Generally, your physician should check your urine every 6 to 12 months for protein excretion. Chapter 5's section on kidney disease explained how a special protein in the urine called albumin may be an early sign that the kidneys are suffering damage. If your urine tests positive for a significant amount of albumin, then you should control your diabetes and blood pressure more tightly, and you may need special medications to protect your kidneys. The good news is that plenty can be done to slow kidney damage. In terms of diet, vegetarian sources of protein might be healthier for the kidney than animal sources. Eating a little less protein or avoiding large amounts of protein in one sitting will protect your kidneys.

Managing My Diabetes Can Be So Overwhelming. How Can I Make Monitoring My Sugar Levels Less of a Burden?

One way to avoid getting overwhelmed with the day-to-day management of diabetes is to break up sugar control into several discrete targets. First, focus on fasting blood sugar in the morning and try to get that under excellent control. Then look at the blood sugars before other meals to see if you can control those. It has been said that if you focus only on the fasting blood sugar control, you won't meet your hemoglobin A1C target of 6.5 percent; perhaps you'll get it down to 7.5 percent or 8 percent. If you really want to get to excellent control, you need to pay attention to what happens to your sugar after eating. Remember, we spend most of our awake time either eating or getting ready for the next meal. By working toward your goals in phases, you can achieve small successes and build on your previous successes. And be prepared for occasional mishaps—accept them, but don't let them hold you back.

Hypoglycemia

The major mishap and perhaps the only mishap we need to be concerned about is hypoglycemia, or low blood sugar, which we discussed in an earlier chapter. We need to recognize the early signs of a low blood sugar level and treat it quickly and appropriately. We also need to know when low blood sugar might occur. Savvy people with diabetes know their bodies and how they respond to various meals, activities, and stresses, and they're good judges of what will happen if a change is implemented. As a patient, pay attention to your body. Watch how different foods affect your sugars, how the timing of your activities might affect your sugars, and how medications affect your sugar levels.

Keeping Tabs on Your Blood Pressure

The goal is to keep your blood pressure below 130/80 mm Hg. To do so, you may need more than one medication. You may also need to see whether you require 24-hour monitoring of your blood pressure to find out if you're experiencing hypertension during the night, which might be harmful. Many of the newer *antihypertension agents* work for 24 hours and are beneficial throughout the day. Just as in the case of blood sugar, you may want to obtain a reliable blood pressure monitor—usually costing in the vicinity of $90 to $100—for home use.

There are several different types of effective blood pressure medications and many research studies have shown that most people need to take 2–3 different blood pressure medications to control their blood pressure. Keeping the blood pressure low has been shown to prevent heart disease, kidney disease and even eye disease.

Keeping Cholesterol Down

Another signpost to look out for on your journey is your cholesterol level. There are a number of different cholesterols, characterized as bad (LDL) cholesterol and good (HDL) cholesterol. Women tend to have higher levels of the good cholesterol than men. For women, HDL should be over 55 mg/dl, and for men, over 45 mg/dl. With LDL cholesterol, however, the motto of the time is "How low can you go?" Just a few years ago, most physicians were satisfied if patients kept their bad cholesterol under 130 mg/dl. Since then, we've realized that it should be less than 100 mg/dl; and many doctors will tell you get all the way down to 80 mg/dl.

If your HDL cholesterol is really low, there's probably not much that will bring it up. A little red wine or lots of exercise or quitting smoking or (for women) taking the female hormone estrogen can elevate the HDL cholesterol. But we can try to lower your LDL cholesterol sufficiently so that the overall ratio of good-to-bad cholesterol is in your favor. And remember that there are lots of excellent cholesterol-lowering medications, so most of us should be able to hit the target.

Practical Tips for Foot Care

Feet can be affected by nerve and/or vascular complications. Neuropathy can show up as tingling or burning at night and later a loss of sensation. If your blood supply is compromised, your feet may feel cold and dry, and your toenails will become thicker and grow slowly. Having poor circulation over a long period of time leads to thin, shiny skin, which can be prone to cuts and infections.

- Often in diabetic neuropathy, a person's feet may be completely numb yet appear pink and warm, as if they still have ample blood flow. This can lull patients into the false belief that they can walk around without shoes. *Never* walk barefoot or in socks, indoors or outdoors, if you can help it.

- Check the tops and bottoms of your feet regularly; ideally before retiring. If it's difficult to see the soles of your feet, try placing a mirror on the floor. You're looking for cracks in the skin or abrasions where you might have cut yourself, as well as calluses, bunions, swelling, or any unusual warmth or change in color.

- Trim your toenails regularly. I have seen nails so long that they curled over and under the toes so that the individual was literally walking on his sharp toenails!

- Choose comfortable shoes. Most foot specialists recommend a good pair of sneakers that offer arch support and can be laced around the ankles. If you have a loss of sensation in the feet, it may be beneficial to wear stiff ankle-length boot-style shoes to help with your walking. And if you're experiencing any changes in the structure of your feet—such as bony abnormalities or unusual pressure points—you may benefit from custom-made shoes. Tip:before putting on your shoes, make sure that there's nothing in them that shouldn't be, like pebbles or little toys that grandchildren will sometimes drop into them.

- Dry, cracked skin can predispose you to infection, so apply a generous amount of moisturizer to your feet every day—ideally, immediately after bathing.

- If you do have an ulcer on the top surface of your foot or on the sole, seek medical attention, regardless of size. Even a seemingly small ulcer can be quite deep and cause major problems. Usually, if you have an ulcer on the bottom of your foot, you should try not to put weight on it. Resting the foot and keeping it elevated will help any medications in the healing process.

Take care of your feet, so that they can take care of you.

Other Things to Watch For

Here are a few more things to do to keep yourself healthy.

- Keeping a diary of your blood sugars, activity levels, and your diet will really let you know what you're doing and how everything affects your sugar control. My five-year-old daughter in prekindergarten has to bring in her "News of the Day" report to the teacher every day. In it, she reports something new or interesting that she's done the previous day. It's hard to believe that with just a little effort, she now has a record of a whole year's worth of activity. It's great to see not only her reflections but also how she's progressed through the year. You can do that with your health as well.

- Think about a door-to-door salesperson. If he'd kept a diary every day of which neighborhoods were more effective, the time of the day sales were better, and which kind of technique was most effective, then he would've done a better job each subsequent month. Likewise for diabetes—by keeping a diary of important factors like sugars, blood pressure, activities, and food intake, you should be able to fine-tune these factors to improve your health. By becoming more self-aware, you'll be better able achieve your goals.

- In addition to the levels you can monitor or the body responses you can keep an eye on, there are other factors that we may not be aware of. These include problems with our eyes, kidneys, cholesterol values, and our heart. For these types of issues, we need to get periodic checkups to find out how things are going. So, at a minimum, you should have your eyes and urine and cholesterol levels checked once a year. The eye checkup may seem to be a bother but, unfortunately, a lot of changes can happen in the back of the eye without our vision being affected immediately. Getting a handle on these changes and treating them early will prevent loss of sight later on. It's important for you to recruit your own professional team of experts. This may include your primary care physician, your endocrinologist, a nurse educator, nutritionist, podiatrist, dentist, and ophthalmologist or optometrist. If it takes a village to raise a child, it almost takes a village to keep someone with diabetes healthy and strong.

The most important thing to remember: *You* are in control. The more seriously you take that role, the happier your life with diabetes can be.

Chapter 7

Diabetes and Nutrition

"**W**e are what we eat." "Food is medicine." You've probably heard these sayings a thousand times. They happen to be true—even more so if you have diabetes.

Our diet consists of carbohydrates, fats, and proteins, along with micronutrients, minerals, and vitamins. Although we pay a lot of attention to carbohydrates, everything on the plate is very important.

Carbohydrates, both simple and complex, are converted to sugar. More than 20 years ago, nutritionists recognized that the amount of carbohydrates in any particular meal has immediate effects on postmeal sugar levels. The amount of fats or proteins does not seem to affect these sugar levels as much. In the long run, however, the type and amount of fats and proteins may affect the development of heart or kidney disease.

After taking everything into account, it is apparent that the *diabetic diet,* explained below, is actually a healthy diet that all of us should follow. Balance, as in all things, is the key.

My Doctor Told Me to Cut My Carbohydrate Intake to No More Than 45 Grams per Meal or within a Four-to-Six-Hour Period. Is That Common Advice for People with Diabetes?

Yes. Diabetes management really boils down to carbohydrate reduction and exercise. And, of course, weight management. Now, this does not mean no carbohydrates at all. If you skip carbohydrates altogether and replace them with fats and proteins, you have to be very careful. Remember that one spoonful of fat has twice the calories of a spoonful of carbohydrates or a spoonful of protein.

Carbs turn into sugar in the body, so eating too many carbs just brings in yet more sugar that has to be moved into the cells. If insulin isn't able to do its job, then the excess sugar winds up lingering in the blood, and up goes your glucose level. Most foods contain carbohydrates, except for protein foods like meat, cheese, eggs, and fats. You don't want to avoid carbs completely, though; you need some sugar to fuel your body. So the idea is to limit them to about 45 grams per day.

The Diabetic Diet: Evolution from Folk Remedy to Science

While a general hypocaloric diet low in sugar has been recommended for hundreds of years, in the 1950s an exchange diet was the fad. The exchange diet allowed you to trade one type of carbohydrate for another. For example, if you wanted to eat a slice of apple pie, you would skip the boiled potato.

A typical unit of carbohydrate contains about 15 grams of carbohydrates. A typical unit of protein is 1 ounce, which may contain 7 grams of protein and 1 to 8 grams of fat, depending on how lean the meat is.

Exchange lists are available for starches, fruits, milk products and meats. So a half cup of pasta is equal to half a hamburger roll is equal to half a bagel is equal to a slice of white bread.

You should note that all milk, whether skim, low fat, or whole, has the same amount of carbohydrates but different amounts of fat. A cup of milk has about 12 grams of carbohydrates.

For fruits, an apple equals:

- Half a nine-inch banana
- 15 grapes
- 1 orange
- 1 small pear
- half cup of pineapple
- 2 plums
- 1 cup of raspberries
- 1¼ cup of strawberries.

One could typically substitute for different meats as well, for beef, pork, poultry or fish, if they are similarly lean.

Remember that a spoonful of fat has twice the calories of a spoonful of protein or carbohydrate. If a portion of meat

Free Foods

You can eat any size portion of the following foods: sugar-free drinks, lettuce, spinach, cabbage, celery, cucumber, green onions, and mushrooms.

is high in fat, it will have far more calories than an extra-lean portion.

• • • *Fast Fact* • • •

Good sources of more information are the American Diabetes Association (*www.diabetes.org*) and the American Dietetic Association (*www.eatright.org*). You can also visit the MayoClinic.com website for easy-to-understand information: *www.mayoclinic.com/ health/diabetes-diet/DA00077.*

• • •

These days, the exchange diet is taught less often. Older diet plans focused on reducing sugar but paid less attention to fat content. Many people with diabetes were unknowingly damaging their arteries and heart with too much dietary fat. So, for example, cereal with skim milk and a sweetener is healthier than cereal with whole milk and no sweetener.

Today's diabetic diet is actually a healthy diet that all people should follow. Approximately 60 percent of total calories can come from carbohydrates, with about 25 percent from protein and the remaining 15 percent from fat. Of the carbohydrates, about 15 percent of your calories can come from simple sugars. Some researchers feel that the amount of carbohydrates should be 40 percent instead of 60 percent. Of course, if you lower your carb intake, you would increase the amounts of protein and/or fat that you eat.

With respect to weight loss, recent research has found that it's the total calories per day that's important rather than the proportion of carbohydrate or fat.

Simple tips to help you get started:

1. Spread your food over three to four meals per day.

2. Increase the amount of fiber in your diet.

3. Pasta or rice serving should be a handful prior to cooking.

4. Reduce the amount of fat, especially, solid fat, in your meals.

5. Meat portions should be about the size of your palm.

6. Use a smaller plate to help with portion control. Half should be vegetables; a quarter should be starch; and a quarter can be vegetarian or meat protein.

7. Use low-fat methods in your cooking.

8. Add lots of color to your meals with vegetables and berries.

9. Do grocery shopping with a list and preferably after having finished a meal.

10. Plan your meals ahead. Call the restaurant ahead, if necessary.

I've Read That Being Overweight Doesn't Cause Diabetes, but Are Overweight People More Likely to Get It?

The short answer is yes—*if* you have the genetic predisposition. Some obese people may never develop diabetes because they don't have the genetic predisposition But if you have both the family history and are overweight, your chances of getting diabetes increase significantly.

Here's how it works:

Your cells need sugar. That's the fuel the brain uses to think, the muscles use to move—all the cells of the body need glucose to do their metabolic work. Insulin transports sugar from the blood into the cells. But a strange thing happens with obese people who are genetically predisposed to diabetes: The more overweight they become, the more the cells become resistant to insulin, and so it takes more and more of the hormone to unlock the cells and get the sugar to them. The exact mechanism isn't completely understood.

People who don't have a genetic predisposition to diabetes can go their whole lives producing more and more insulin and getting it into the cells, and so their blood sugars stay down. But in a person who has a predisposition to diabetes, the pancreas doesn't function normally. There's a defect. What happens is that eventually the organ can't go on producing insulin year after year after year. After a while, it starts scaling back, and blood sugars rise.

My Doctor Told Me to Eat Lots of Vegetables— Don't They Have Carbohydrates, Too?

It's true that some vegetables contain carbohydrates, but they don't have much. Some vegetables contain very, very little; it depends on the vegetable. However, we still recommend that diabetes patients introduce more vegetables into their diets because they fill you up and are low in calories. They're really ideal for diabetes, especially if you're trying to lose weight.

Most nutritionists recommend that you fill half your plate with vegetables if you're trying to lose weight and watch your blood sugar.

Is It Okay to Fill Up on Other Noncarb Foods That Are High in Protein but Low in Sugar, Like Cheese or Peanut Butter?

Cheese and peanut butter fill you up and have protein, but they're also laden with fat. High-fat foods are heart unhealthy, plus they won't help you lose weight. However, some types of fat (in moderation) are less harmful than others.

Peanut butter, for example, is high in calories, but at least it's a healthy fat. Cheese, on the other hand, is full of saturated fat, which is very unhealthy and should be eaten in very limited amounts.

I Feel So Limited in What I Can Eat, and Nothing That I'm Supposed to Eat Seems to Fill Me Up. How Can I Deal with My Hunger?

If you're following the prescribed diabetic diet and find that you're hungry much of the time, try adding more fiber to your diet. Fiber helps keep you full longer. *Soluble fiber,* like oat fiber or psyllium, even has cholesterol-reducing benefits.

Most fiber-rich foods have both soluble fiber and *insoluble fiber,* so you just want to think high fiber in general. Whole grains such as brown rice and oats benefit you, while breads, pastas, and other products made from whole wheat are going to keep you full longer and help you to eat less.

I Want to Be Healthy, but It's So Hard to Change My Eating Habits. How Do You Motivate Yourself to Eat Right?

Your doctor may refer you to a nutritionist or diet specialist who will help you manage your diabetes diet. He or she will likely begin by conducting a nutrition assessment, to obtain an accurate diet history from you, identify the foods you like, and then "negotiate" which foods you're willing to give up or cut down on. Together you'll try to incorporate the diet into your current eating habits rather than attempting a complete overhaul. Not only is that unnecessary (unless you've been living on nothing but, say, Twinkies and coconut syrup), but the majority of folks wouldn't stick to a radically different dietary plan, at least not for long.

Some people truly want to be told exactly what to eat, but they're definitely in the minority. A good nutritionist will help you see that making small adjustments here and there can add up to make a big difference.

Is It Safe for Me to Diet to Help Me Lose Weight?

Weight Watchers, NutriSystem, Jenny Craig, and a few others weight-loss programs are extremely sensible. Again, the trend in diets is moving more toward personal choices and away from rigid eating plans that no one likes and many find difficult to follow.

Ideally, a weight-loss program should teach you how to eat a well-balanced diet that you can follow for the rest of your life. Most diets are temporary "fad" diets—they're not meant to be lifelong eating plans.

Your local diabetes education program or your hospital's nutrition department may also offer healthy nutrition programs and weight-loss programs.

How Much Protein Is Too Much? Is the Limit Different for People with Diabetes?

For a healthy person, with or without diabetes, 0.8 grams of protein per kilogram of body weight (that's roughly 2.2 pounds) is plenty. Very, *very* few men and women in this country don't meet their protein requirements. The only people for whom it might be a challenge to consume adequate protein would be those who are ill and just can't bring themselves to eat, or someone with increased protein needs, like a burn patient or a kidney dialysis patient. Most Americans actually get two to three times their daily protein requirements.

If you have early kidney failure due to diabetes, further restriction of protein intake may be beneficial in slowing down the decline in kidney function.

Protein isn't only, or even mainly, found in meat, it's in many of the things we eat routinely, such as milk, starches (breads, cereals, pastas), and even fruits and vegetables.

Should I Focus on Carbs and Not Worry So Much about Fat in My Diet?

Anyone trying to lose weight has to be concerned about fat, because fat is very high in calories. Fat has 9 calories per gram, whereas 1 gram of carbohydrates has only 4.5 calories a gram, and 1 gram of protein, 4 calories. But most protein foods also contain a lot of fat, which raises its calorie level. The easiest way to cut the calories in your diet is to cut the fat.

On a very low-fat diet, people tend to eat more because they're hungry all the time; fat tends to be filling because it's harder to digest and takes longer for your body to process. Therefore, a little fat can actually help you, preventing you from eating more between meals or at the next meal.

Should I Be Adding Olive Oil to All My Food to Increase My Intake of "Healthy" Fats?

No. Olive oil has just as many calories as any other fat.

Do I Have to Watch My Sodium, Too?

Everyone should limit his or her sodium, but it's especially important for people with diabetes, who face a higher than average risk of heart disease.

The typical American eats 3,000 to 5,000 milligrams of sodium a day, with many people consuming even more than that. However, endurance athletes (exercising for more than two hours) have increased sodium requirements due to excessive sweat losses. Hypertensive individuals are recommended to limit their sodium intake to less than 2,400 milligrams daily, along with eating a low-fat diet rich in fruits, vegetables, whole grains, and low-fat dairy foods, as part of blood pressure management.

The 2005 dietary guidelines for people with hypertension calls for less than 2,300 milligrams a day, and for African-Americans, less than 1,500 milligrams a day. To give you a guideline, one teaspoon of salt contains 2,300 milligrams. But that doesn't mean you can add that amount to your food, because there's already sodium in food naturally. Only about 5 percent to 10 percent of our daily sodium intake should come from a salt shaker. Common dietary sources of sodium are often processed foods to which salt is added during preparation, such as cheeses, soups, pickles, and pretzels. Also, commercially prepared foods or restaurant foods are generally high in sodium.

The table below will give you an idea of the relative amounts of sodium in various foods.

Table 2. Sodium Content of Food

Food	Sodium (mg)
Table salt, 1 tsp	2,358
Dill pickle, 1 large	1,731
Canned chicken soup, 1 cup	850
Sauerkraut, ½ cup	780
Pretzels, 1 oz	486
Cottage cheese, ½ cup	459
Deli ham, 1 oz	341
Deli turkey breast, 1 oz	335
Soy sauce, 1 tsp	304
American cheese, 1 oz	304
Cornflakes, 1 cup	298
Deli bologna,	295
Potato chips, 1 oz	183

How Does Alcohol Affect Diabetes?

Many people forget that liquids have nutritional values, too. Alcohol contains calories, and those calories add up. For someone who's not on a hypoglycemic medication, alcohol may have modest effects. But a person taking a glucose-lowering agent or insulin must drink with caution. Too much alcohol can also make it more difficult for you to sense a low blood sugar, since you'll be unsure if the lightheadedness or other symptoms are from that or from the alcohol. Incidentally, the dietary guidelines classify wine, beer, and hard liquor equally.

Should I Avoid Trans Fats?

Only since 2006 has the FDA required food manufacturers to list trans fats on products' Nutrition Facts labels. Trans-fatty acids are often oils with hydrogen atoms added to make them solid, or "spreadable." They last for a long time in the body and may accelerate hardening of the arteries. An example is margarine. When comparing products, simply add the amounts (in grams) of trans fat and saturated fat together, and choose the one with the lowest total.

I See Foods Labeled "Reduced Fat," "Low Fat," and "No Fat"—Is There a Big Difference?

Yes. The least impressive claim is "reduced fat." It's the one you see most at the supermarket, though, because it's the easiest of the three to manufacture. Reduced fat tells you that the product contains at least 25 percent less fat than the original. That's not the same as low fat.

For example, most people think that 2 percent milk is low fat. It's not. If you look on the label, it says "reduced fat." The next level of fat reduction would be "light," which means one-third fewer calories, or half the fat of the original. So that's a little better than reduced. If you look at "low fat," it's actually a measurable amount—3 grams or less of fat per serving—as opposed to a percentage based on something else. Think of it this way: Something that's extremely high in fat, like butter or margarine, is maybe 97 percent fat; 25 percent less than 97 percent is still is a lot of fat! Light margarine is usually one-half the fat. That's impressive. But low fat, at 3 grams or less, truly is low. As for "fat free," it too is a measurable quantity: less than a half gram of fat per serving. So here's the order of preferences, from best to worst: fat free, low fat, light, and reduce.

How Does Serving Size Come into Play?

Many labels can be misleading if you don't pay attention to the serving size as defined by the product's manufacturer. To make things even more confusing, companies constantly change what constitutes a serving to better suit their marketing needs. An example of that would be what they did with yogurt. The typical yogurt container used to be eight ounces; now they've made a serving six ounces. Next time you're in a grocery store, take a look at the label for a "low-carb" single-serving frozen entrée; it may have a low amount of carbs in it, but if the serving size is actually half a box, then you have to double all the nutritional values to see what you're really eating. This is a common trick: If a company wants to make something "low-carb" or "low-cal," it will halve the normal serving size so that a single-serving meal actually contains two servings, nutritionally speaking. You have to read really carefully.

What's Better for Me: Sugar-Free Ice Cream or Fat-Free Ice Cream?

Fat-free ice cream is better for you than sugar-free ice cream that's not fat free. Why? Because ice cream that's not fat-free contains saturated fat—an animal fat, and very heart unhealthy. If it's fat free but not sugar free, you can still work it into your carb allotment. Sugar can be incorporated into your diet in healthy ways; saturated fat shouldn't be included at all.

You have to watch those so-called low-carb ice creams too, because a lot of them contain sugar alcohols, which raise blood sugar. They're listed on the label, but the manufacturers subtract them from the total number of carbs. Tip: Never go by "Net Carbs," because that's not a government-regulated term.

Such unregulated terms can be whatever the manufacturer wants it to be. For example, one brand of "low-carb" ice cream has 20 grams of sugar alcohol in one serving, but it subtracted that full 20 grams out of the total carbs and came up with this really low net carb figure. But, really, you have to take the sugar alcohol number and count it at about half the rate, then add it to the total carb figure; so 10 grams of that should have been left in. So now we're back to an ice cream that, as far as people with diabetes are concerned, has a lot of carbs.

The people who really get into this kind of calculation are men and women on *insulin-to-carb ratios,* for which they take

Tip

With the zero-calorie sugar substitute sucralose (Splenda), you can cook or bake just as you would with regular sugar. The artificial sweetener aspartame (NutraSweet, Equal) breaks down at high temperatures, diminishing its sweetness.

so many units of insulin for so many grams of carbohydrates. Most people with diabetes don't need to do this. Unless you are dosing your insulin to your carbohydrates, you really just need to count the total carbs.

With So Many Conflicting Diet Messages Out There, I've Gotten Very Confused. What Kind of Overall Diet Is Best?

Some diets, like the Atkins diet, will tell you that fat is okay as long as your carbs are low, but the recommendation for all Americans is to follow a low-fat diet—that doesn't mean very low fat, it just means generally low fat, or no more than 30 percent of your daily calories. However, for someone with diabetes, it's even more important because he or she is more at risk for heart disease.

Chapter 8

Exercising without (Much) Pain

People who define exercise as moving their arms and legs so they arrive at the same place as they began—moving but not going anywhere—probably think that exercise is a futile waste of energy. Centuries ago, and even as recently as 75 years ago, we toiled for our food, and everything we did in life required manual labor. To get water for the family required a walk to the town well and bringing back buckets of water. Getting our food meant daily trips to the market or harvesting from our own gardens, fields, and small farms. In most cultures, organized sport was not available—in fact, it was unnecessary. People were active with their daily needs, so exercise was life and life was exercise.

Today, as we rush from one appointment to another, pick up the dry cleaning, work at a desk for ten hours, courier our children from place to place, and finally collapse at the end of the day, we find ourselves with no time to exercise. For most people, exercise is like the least favorite relative on your gift list. And, of course, if you exercise (or plan to exercise) by yourself, you can always postpone it to another time, because you only have to deal with your own schedule, whereas when you exercise with a friend or spouse, you are obligated to show up—and to exercise.

Incorporating Exercise into Your Day— Painlessly

So how can we incorporate exercise into our daily lives without it being a pain in the neck (or anywhere else)? Here are 24 tips that will help.

1. Park your car as far as you can from your workplace. You have to get to work anyway, so this is a necessary movement, and you don't need to think of it as exercise.

2. Park your car as far as you safely can when you go shopping. How often do you drive around and around the parking lot at a grocery or department store trying to find that ideal parking spot next to the main entrance? In fact, parking your car at the most remote corner of the parking lot and then walking to the main entrance is often quicker than

driving around hunting for that spot. But do be mindful of safety concerns, and make sure that you park in a well-lit area.

3. Walk to your grocery or drugstore instead of driving. Take a cart or a bicycle with a basket. The best thing about walking *to* a destination is that you also have to walk *back,* so it doubles the amount of exercise.

4. Develop a buddy system for whichever exercise activity you plan to get into, be it bicycling, tennis, badminton, bowling, golf, whatever. Making appointments with friends will force you to commit, and small group activities are always more practical.

5. Larger group activities are more difficult to organize, but this ups the ante for you to be committed. Join a local softball or basketball league, or organize pickup games between friends at home or at work. Because you're part of a team, you'll want to be responsible and show up and be active. This is a good way to build friendships, exercise, and have fun at the same time.

6. At work, take the stairs instead of the elevator. One nurse in my department was claustrophobic—she was afraid to get into an elevator, so she always took the stairs. She didn't seem too happy about this at first, but she became very fit!

7. Some of my colleagues actually run to work—maybe five miles or so—take a shower, do their work, and then run back (or sometimes hitch a ride with another colleague). This allows them to exercise as part of their daily routine.

8. If you have to drive, try to do some isometric exercises of your stomach, thighs, legs and feet, and occasionally your arms, without jeopardizing your safety. Isometric exercises call for tightening and relaxing your muscles without actually moving any limbs. You tighten your muscles for ten seconds, then relax for ten seconds, and then repeat this cycle at least ten times. Do these exercises when you're on a plane, too. Your chances of developing a blood clot in your legs are substantially higher when you're in a seated position for a long time. You can minimize this risk by exercising in place.

9. If you're working at your desk, do the above iso-metric exercises, and stretch and push your arms against the desk and perform leg-strengthening exercises as well. When you're on the phone (unless it's a video phone), the caller never needs to know that you're stretching and exercising while you're talking (unless you start grunting and groaning).

10. When sitting at your desk or on a plane, try not to cross your legs for too long a time. This can lead to an increased tendency to develop blood clots in your legs, and these can be potentially dangerous.

11. If you go out for lunch, walk to the restaurant instead of driving. This will allow you to burn some calories, which will offset some of the calories you take in while eating.

12. When you take your children to their soccer or base-ball games, don't just sit there and yell at the coach

or referee. While your daughter is playing soccer or your son is playing tennis, walk around the park or soccer field for a half hour. You'll get some pleasant exercise and work off any steam generated at your job (or by your kid's team's performance on the field). The bonus here is that you know where your children are, your children are getting exercise, and you'll be getting a workout, too.

13. If you use a treadmill or a stationary bicycle at home, watch the news or listen to an audiobook. This kind of multitasking doesn't induce stress (well, depending on what's being reported on the news) and allows you to enjoy the exercise without thinking of it as exercise. These days, many cruise ships have exercise facilities, and there's nothing more wonderful than running on a treadmill with a beautiful view of the ocean and listening to music.

14. Get a pedometer, note how many steps you take per day, and then try to increase the number by 10 percent each week. Try to get to at least 5,000 steps per day. This is a cheap way to really document how many steps you're taking. It also tells you how active you are at work. Most of us think we're much more active at work than we really are. Keeping a log of your progress is a good motivational tool. Don't worry about the number so much, but look at how many steps you're taking now and then, slowly trying to increase the number of steps every day. (And please don't cheat the system by attaching the pedometer to your dog.)

15. If you enjoy your morning coffee and newspaper, walk to the local coffee shop to get the paper and coffee. It will be a win-win scenario, and you won't feel like you did all that walking for nothing. Perhaps at the coffee shop you'll meet some regular customers with whom you'll discuss politics or sports (or exercising). Maybe you'll meet a walking partner.

16. Try to eat standing up. When you stand, you expend more calories, and thus you'll also be able to eat a little more. You may actually be more comfortable eating while standing.

17. Put weights around your ankles and do leg bends or knee bends while you watch television or work on the computer. The added weight will strengthen your muscles and improve your bone density.

18. When you do a household activity such as vacuuming, cleaning, or gardening, a TV will imprison you, whereas a radio, an MP3 player, a Walkman, or an iPod will give you more freedom to move about. I remember getting my first TV shortly after moving to Boston, and I quickly noticed that with the television on I was stuck—I wouldn't leave the room—whereas with the radio or music playing, I was quite mobile and could do other household chores.

19. During the winter, go to the shopping mall and leave your money at home. Go before the stores open and get in your exercise by walking around the mall in a safe, heated environment. Many

shopping malls have walking clubs that meet before the stores open.

20. Don't just watch your children dance. Start an adult folk-dancing club or take up the waltz, cha-cha, or fox-trot. Dancing is great exercise, improving your cardiac fitness without overstraining the heart.

21. Mow your own lawn. Save money and improve your health.

22. When you organize family outings, try to incorporate outdoor games into the activities. Work in skiing, baseball, Frisbee, cricket, or badminton, rather than just eating and drinking. This is good for group interactions: It will increase bonding among cousins and improve everyone's health.

23. If you travel out of town for meetings, talk to the hotel concierge and get tips on safe local walking tours or jogging routes. Too often, when we travel, we end up seeing only the hotel and the airport before returning home. You miss out on the whole reason why those meetings were held at these places. Get out and enjoy the scenery and, as they say, smell the roses.

24. If you want to feel more energetic after eating, avoid alcohol or high-fat and high-carbohydrate foods. Eat more vegetables and fruits and increase your fiber intake. Heavy meats, alcohol, and high-fat foods are harder to digest and are more likely to slow you down.

For diabetes, exercise is like a medication. Exercising just two to four times a week has great benefits and improves insulin's efficiency in getting those sugars into your muscle tissue. Stop exercising, and within three to four days, your body will become more insulin resistant, and you may find that your sugars will sneak up on you.

Besides improving blood sugar control in most people with type 2 diabetes, exercise may help lower bad cholesterol, raise good cholesterol, enhance well-being, result in weight loss, and improve overall cardiac health. Yet exercise is one of the most difficult things to get people to do—even when their lives literally depend on it. Unfortunately, Lisa Linder had to witness this strange psychology at work in her own family.

Lisa has had type 1 diabetes for nearly 40 years—since she was 10. She has seen and experienced all of the changing ideas, beliefs, practices, and innovations regarding diabetes, and *a lot* has changed in those 40 years. She has some pretty firm beliefs of her own as well.

Lisa's Story

When I was about ten years old, I put on quite a bit of weight, and I was constantly hungry, constantly thirsty. And then, all of sudden, even though I was continuing to eat and drink a lot, the weight began melting off of me. I went from ninety-eight pounds to sixty-eight pounds in two months. My clothes were falling off, and my mother couldn't figure out what was going on. I told her I felt shaky all the time, but I couldn't describe what "shaky" meant. She took me to several doctors, and they said, "Oh, she just lost her baby fat; it's fine, don't worry about it."

They weren't alarmed, like they would be today. She took me to the Cleveland Clinic, where they did a blood sugar test. They took a tube of blood, and I wasn't allowed to go home. They said, "She's checking in." And back then, you checked in for a week.

I don't know what my glucose number was, but we were told that I was within two weeks of going into a coma, that's how high it was. It probably was seven hundred to nine hundred. When it's that high for that long a period of time, some really serious problems can develop. That's why you end up going into a coma from high sugar.

I had no family history of diabetes, but the doctors contended that a childhood illness like measles, mumps, or chicken pox had settled in my pancreas. That was their presumption back then. They may have different ideas about it today, but no one else in our family had diabetes until my father developed adult-onset diabetes later.

When they sent me home, I was on one insulin shot a day. The only way to know what your blood sugar was back then was to either go to the doctor and have three or four blood tests or check your urine, but that's not accurate, because if your sugar is under control, you don't urinate as much. If your sugar is out of control, you'll go to the bathroom more frequently, but that's the nature of your body, trying to eliminate the sugar.

I checked my urine four to six times a day, and it got confusing, because sometimes my sugar count just felt low, and I got the cold sweats and this jittery, shaky feeling, but yet my urine was telling me that my sugar count was high. So it's not a foolproof method, because the urine could've been sitting inside my body for however many hours before I went, and then the count wouldn't be accurate. It was a really bad, bad situation; I never really knew what the count was unless I went in and had my blood tested.

When they finally developed blood glucose monitoring machines—I was about eighteen or nineteen then—it created a whole new life for diabetics: to be able to know almost instantaneously where your blood sugar was. And as a type 1 diabetic, I could always get the insulin to bring my sugar down if it was too high.

Today I test my blood sugar four to six times a day. It's a hard thing to get used to, but in many ways, I think it might be easier for juvenile diabetics like me, because this is a way of life for me. I've done this since I was ten, and I think that people who have to start all this stuff as adults have a harder time getting into the habit of doing it. So the longer you have diabetes, the easier it is. The complications are inevitable, but I've been a firm believer that with the help of the man upstairs and trying my very best to take care of myself, so far, knock on wood, I'm doing okay. I had a little bit of laser treatment in one eye, but other than that I've been fine.

I have my eyes examined twice a year, and my eyes have shown no more deterioration. I'm actually quite fine. I was also in a kidney study for four years, about ten years ago, for these inhibitor drugs in diabetics and did very well with that too—no kidney damage that I'm aware of.

After I got on insulin, my weight leveled off; I really have never been ultraheavy. I could probably stand to lose ten or fifteen pounds at this point, but during my teen years I was fine. I was just always right around 115 or 120 pounds, and I'm five-foot-six.

I was told to exercise. But I was also told to watch how much I exercised because of the fact that when you're on insulin shots, you have to be very routine oriented. You've got to try to do the same things every day. And in school, you have gym class on Mondays, Wednesdays, and Fridays, so my gym teachers always had to be on the lookout to see if I was walking around looking like I was a little dazed or confused. Or if my sugar was low, they knew to give me some orange juice right away.

I've always tried to be somewhat active, though I don't strenuously exercise. Right now I ride a Cardio Glide several times a week for a half hour, and my dog loves long walks, so on weekends my husband and I take her out on a two- or three-mile walk, and we walk at a pretty brisk pace.

Now I have the insulin pump. It's a twofold method. You need to be very mathematical in using an insulin pump, because you're doing several things with the device. It's always giving me a minute amount of insulin, called a basal rate. It's giving me 0.6 units every hour, and every three minutes it's giving me a very small amount of insulin—it works the same way that a normal person's pancreas works.

The pump doesn't really get in the way of anything. I unhook it for ten minutes every day to take a shower, and as soon as I get out of the shower, I plug it back in. It's unplugged, but the other part is still inside of me.

The pump is a great success. I've been on it for about two and a half years, and I have to say that I'd trade in my husband before I'd trade in the pump. I mean, it's created a whole new life for me. Prior to this, I was on five or six shots a day. When I was a teenager, I went from one shot to two shots a day; then when I was in my early- to mid-twenties, I went to four shots a day; and in my early forties, I went to five or six shots a day. Now the pump does all of that automatically for me.

Really, all things considered, my life is pretty good now. I feel great. But it was a long road. And, sadly, though my experiences may serve as an example to others of how to manage their diabetes, I really hoped that my father would have known better to learn from my trials. It's interesting how folks often look after others better than they do themselves.

My father was not the most compliant person with diabetes. In a lot of ways, since I've been diabetic longer—even though I've got a better chance of having these complications set in—I know enough to try really hard to do what's right most of the time. That gives me more of a chance to carry on with this disease for a longer period of time than someone who's trying to learn to change their old, comfortable habits.

I've always been a firm believer in seeing a specialist for whatever your problem is. I've been seeing an endocrinologist since I was ten. And that was thirty-eight years ago. I'm very thankful for all the progress that's been made in endocrinology and diabetes research, and all of the wonderful medications and equipment they've come up with for diabetics to live more normal lives and keep them healthier longer. It's much easier to live with this disease today than twenty or thirty years ago. The changes I've seen in my lifetime have been astounding.

Some Words of Caution

Men and women with type 1 diabetes can benefit from exercise, but it may not improve your blood sugar control. In fact, if you're not careful, sometimes exercise can worsen glucose control, with lots of low sugars or high sugars. When you exercise, your muscles rely on glucose for energy. When you stop, your muscles are still metabolically very active. They continue to consume more glucose and accept more sugar from the blood. So patients who have type 1 diabetes or who are on insulin therapy may find that their sugars drop several hours after they exercise. This can be prevented by adjusting the insulin or eating the right number of calories.

Another concern about physical activity is that if you overdo it, you may increase the amount of adrenaline and other hormones in your blood that would elevate your sugar significantly.

Overall, however, exercise is still very important in the management of diabetes. You just need to pay attention to your body and take certain precautions, as with many other aspects of your life.

Not all exercise is for everyone. Some of us like to ski, some of us like to play tennis, and some of us like to bike.

Move to Improve

1. Start slow. If you haven't been active in a long time, check with your doctor before you begin.

2. Increase your activity minutes day by day. Plan a daily calendar, penciling in your goal minutes per day.

3. Do something you enjoy.

4. Enhance your environment. Go to the park. Take your favorite music. Listen to an audiobook. Take a friend. This is one of the few areas of life where we can truly multitask.

5. Try to get at least 150 minutes of activity per week.

6. If you walk, pretend that you're walking across the country. Pretty soon, you'll be crossing the state line!

7. Check your sugars before and after your activity. Know how your body responds.

8. Generally, it's better to be active after a meal.

9. As you become increasingly active, you may need to adjust your medications downward.

10. Never give up! If for some reason you have to stop, don't be disheartened. Always pick yourself up and start moving again.

Before you embark on a formal exercise program, it's important to get a medical evaluation—especially if you're older and haven't exercised in a number of years.

Certain complications of diabetes will dictate what kinds of exercises you can do. For example, if you have problems with neuropathy and poor sensation in your feet, running isn't a good choice, whereas swimming might be very helpful. If you have retinopathy, then you might not want to lift weights, because the stress could possibly injure the fragile blood vessels in the back of the eye. Ideally, tailor your physical activity to your background, interests, and the types of complications you might have.

It may also be necessary to adjust your medications. In general, I advise people to exercise after eating, to reduce the risk of hypoglycemia. Also try to exercise at around the same time every day, so that you can see a pattern and modify your meals or medications accordingly.

With respect to insulin, you may need to reduce the amount of fast-acting insulin that you take prior to exercise. This is highly individual: Some people can skip an entire dose, whereas others may need to reduce their insulin by 50 percent or so. If you're taking a pill that could lower your blood sugar, you may need to either delay the medication or cut the dose in half. Ask your doctor if your pills increase pancreatic insulin secretion. Pills called *insulin sensitizers* usually don't cause low blood sugars related to exercise.

No matter what you decide to do, it's always important to check your glucose more often around the time of exercise to ensure that your sugar is not going too high or too low.

Let's get going! I'll see you outside.

Chapter 9

Combat: Medicines That Fight Diabetes

M any medicines are available to people with type 2 diabetes. But before we examine them, let's quickly review the causes of high blood sugars. Perhaps you're absorbing the sugars very rapidly from your stomach. Or your pancreas isn't making enough insulin to drive the blood sugar into your fat and muscle, resulting in a backup and high concentrations of glucose in the blood. Another possibility is that your body is making plenty of insulin but can't seem to use the hormone effectively. Lately, scientists theorize that levels of the "anti-insulin" hormone glucagon may be higher in type 2 diabetes.

Here's how the different medications work in your body:

- By slowing down the rate at which sugar is absorbed from your stomach.

- By stimulating the pancreas to release more insulin from the Beta cells.

- By suppressing your glucagon levels from the alpha cells in the pancreas.

- By enhancing insulin's effectiveness.

Remember, your blood sugar level reflects how much glucose is being made or released into the bloodstream, balanced against how efficiently your tissues use this fuel.

Now let's take a look at the various ways we try to combat the causes of diabetes.

Drugs: Your Weapons against Diabetes

If you read about the history of drugs and therapies for diabetes, you may find lots of curious choices. Before much was known about the science of diabetes, all sorts of substances had been proposed—from arsenic, to chromium, to zinc, to herbs such as cinnamon, aloe vera, and many others.

In the modern age, we have evolved from medications that stimulate the beta cells in the pancreas to medications that improve how insulin works. More recently, new drugs that work by other mechanisms have become available, such as drugs that slow down glucose absorption from the gut and a cholesterol-lowering drug that also lowers blood sugar

Meds Aren't the Total Answer

When taking any medication for diabetes, it's essential to follow a healthy lifestyle of good nutrition and exercise. *That is the cornerstone of treatment.* Before taking any medication, discuss the benefits and risks with your physician. You cannot afford to be a silent partner.

levels. There is also a new pill that increases the levels of certain hormones; these in turn instruct the beta cells to increase insulin production in response to rising sugar levels and order the alpha cells to make less glucagon.

What are some trends?

The oldest drugs we have at our disposal typically can lower sugar levels below normal at times (hypoglycemia). This is probably because insulin release can occur even when the sugars are dropping.

Newer drugs are less likely to cause hypoglycemia by themselves. In this scenario, when the sugar levels are falling, insulin release is also falling.

Another desired characteristic is durability. We know that with type 2 diabetes, the pancreas's beta cells eventually fail. It would be valuable to have drugs that can maintain healthy beta cells for many years.

Antidiabetic Agents

Alpha-glucosidase inhibitors (acarbose, miglitol). Acarbose (brand name: Precose) and miglitol (Glyset) affect how we absorb sugars from the stomach and gut. Most of the carbohydrates in our diet are broken down to sugar molecules joined in pairs. These pairs must then be broken down into individual sugar molecules in order for our small intestine to absorb them. Acarbose and miglitol inhibit this process by interfering with a crucial enzyme. As you might guess, it's important to take these medications before you eat. Both acarbose and miglitol are fairly effective at reducing high blood sugars after a meal.

When those paired blood sugars aren't adequately absorbed as they travel through your small and large intestines, they can cause diarrhea and gas. Although these side effects might make for cocktail party humor, they tend to subside once you've been taking either medication for a while. You might think about using these medications for weight loss, but studies have shown that they are not effective in that regard, perhaps because the sugar is still being absorbed but at a far slower rate, or we're substituting fat for sugar and carbohydrates—and that, of course, defeats the purpose of taking the medication in the first place.

Sulfonylureas (chlorpropamide, glyburide, glipizide, glimepiride). This class of medication, which stimulates the pancreas to release more insulin in response to high blood sugars, is the oldest of the modern era of antidiabetic agents. Soon after World War II, when research was being performed on newer antibiotics, some of these sulfa-derivative components were found to have a sugar lowering effect. This is how chlorpropamide (brand name: Diabinese), the first sulfonylurea, or SFU for short, was discovered. These pills appeared to improve insulin secretion. Sometimes, though, they caused the blood sugars to fall below normal and thus were called oral hypoglycemic agents.

Chlorpropamide has unusual side effects: Some patients who drank alcohol after taking the medication would become extremely flushed. Very rarely, a minority of people registered a low sodium level, which altered their mental faculties. And sometimes in elderly patients whose kidneys were functioning at half speed, the drug and its metabolites built up in the body and caused prolonged hypoglycemia.

Over the years, safer cousins of chlorpropamide have been developed and are widely used: glyburide (Micronase, Diabeta), glipizide (Glucotrol), and glimepiride (Amaryl). These drugs interact with special receptors on pancreatic beta cells—like keys turning on a car's ignition—and spur the cells to secrete insulin. A frequent potential side effect is hypoglycemia, which can occasionally be prolonged. So it's important for you to vigilantly monitor your eating and exercise habits.

Meglitinides (repaglinide, nateglinide). These two new medications aren't sulfa derivatives, but they interact with the SFU receptors on pancreatic cells to release insulin. Repaglinide (brand name: Prandin) and nateglinide (Starlix) are short acting and must be taken before each meal. They appear to be less likely than SFUs to cause low blood sugars. They can also be taken if someone's kidneys are functioning at only about 40 percent.

Dipeptidyl Peptidase-4 (DPP-4) inhibitors (sitagliptin). Did you know that when you drink a sugary beverage, it will actually cause a better insulin response from your pancreas than if you were to give yourself an injection of intravenous sugar?

That's because after years of research, we now know that the stomach and the gut are large hormone-producing organs. When food enters your stomach, it begins a virtual symphony of hormone release from your stomach and your small intestine. One group of hormones is called *incretins,* because they increase the secretion of insulin from the pancreas.

The two major incretins are GLP-1 (glucagonlike-peptide 1) and GIP (glucose-dependent insulinotropic peptide). Of note, GLP-1 also appears to reduce the amount of glucagon, insulin's hormonal opposite. (You may recall that glucagon elevates blood sugar levels.) Compared to people who don't have diabetes, people with type 2 diabetes appear to have lower blood levels of GLP-1 and less effective GIP.

A new oral medication, sitagliptin (Januvia), boosts levels of both GLP-1 and GIP by blocking the action of DPP-4 enzymes, which quickly break down incretins. This results in improved insulin secretion in response to changes in glucose and improved blood sugars. When used alone or with metformin or a TZD, low blood sugars have not been a problem. Also, sitagliptin is thought to be relatively weight neutral. You should watch for any episodes of colds or sore throat or headaches, and for any type of allergic reaction. If you already have kidney problems, your doctor may decide to use a lower dose of the medication. Other DPP-4 inhibitors are being actively developed in the U.S. and abroad.

Biguanides (metformin). Metformin (Glucophage) has been available in the United States since 1994 and in the rest of the world for more than 45 years, yet we still haven't figured out exactly how it works. However, we do know that the oral drug doesn't increase insulin secretion from the pancreas and therefore doesn't cause hypoglycemia. It appears to cut down the amount of sugar produced by the liver, as well as decrease the body's insulin resistance; therefore, metformin may help reduce early morning high blood sugars. It may also cut your appetite and facilitate your ability to lose weight. Side effects include gas and diarrhea, and patients should take the medication with food. The typical dose varies between 1,000 milligrams and 2,500 milligrams per day.

Rarely, when people with liver or kidney disease or with unstable heart failure take metformin, they may increase their risk of developing *lactic acidosis,* a serious condition where lactic acid accumulates in the blood. If you have ever experienced severe muscle cramps with extreme exercise, it may have been due to a buildup of lactic acid. As with any medication, one needs to use the right amount of medication for the right person.

• • • *Fast Fact* • • •

Metformin does not cause liver or kidney disease.
However, if you already have significant liver or
kidney disease, you should *not* take metformin.

• • •

Thiazolidinediones (TZDs) (rosiglitazone, pioglitazone).
Thiazolidenediones (TZDs) work at the level of the nucleus,

which is the brain center for each one of your cells. These pills lower blood sugar by enhancing insulin's effect on fat and muscle tissue, so that the sugar enters cells more easily. You may not see an effect for several weeks, so be patient. It has been suggested that thiazolidenediones may allow you to control your blood glucose levels longer than older medications like metformin and sulfonylureas.

Side effects may include fluid retention, swollen ankles, and weight gain. Some patients find that they have less swelling when they take these medications at night. Women tend to respond better than men to TZDs. Of course, women have more body fat compared to men, and fat tissue is one of the medications' targets.

Rosiglitazone (Avandia) and pioglitazone (Actos) are currently the available TZDs. These medications shouldn't be taken by people who have experienced heart failure, and should be used with caution by other patients. People with congestive heart failure, where the heart doesn't pump efficiently, or those who are already on insulin therapy, are likely to retain fluid and experience swelling, which can be counteracted by using a water pill, or diuretic. If you have heart failure, TZDs are not for you.

These medications may have a beneficial effect on the fats in the blood.

Recently, there has been some concern about the drugs' effects on bone. TZDs may cause some thinning of the bone around the wrist-hand and ankle-foot areas. This is especially so in older women. Although only a few people may report fractures in these areas, if you are older or have osteoporosis, you should check with your doctor. She may be able to devise a regimen to reduce your risk.

Red Flag

People who have diabetes and either liver disease or moderate heart failure should not take TZDs. There may be extenuating circumstances. So always discuss with your physician.

Rosiglitazone had been in the media a lot because a preliminary analysis of older data suggested that patients treated with it may have a higher risk of a cardiac event. However, this has not been confirmed by more recent studies. Remember, you do need to manage your blood pressure and cholesterol to reduce your risk of heart disease. However, if you're about to start on a TZD therapy, then your doctor needs to assess your diabetes and your risk of heart disease, and then decide which agent might be more suitable for you.

Cholesterol reducers (colesevelam). Colesevelam (Welchol), actually a cholesterol lowering drug, can reduce blood sugar levels in patients with type 2 diabetes mellitus when added to other antidiabetic medications (metformin, sulfonylureas, or insulin). Since colesevelam works primarily in your gut, you might anticipate some stomach side effects.

Tell your doctor if you have digestive problems, including gastroparesis (in which the stomach takes too long to empty), abnormal contractions of the GI tract, trouble swallowing, and vitamin A, D, E, or K deficiencies, or if you've had major gastrointestinal surgery.

The usual regimen of six tablets per day should be taken about four hours away from other medications.

Hormonal Therapy

Insulin. The body makes tiny amounts of insulin even when we're not eating, to keep things at an even keel. When we eat, insulin surges to meet the rising blood sugar and bring it down nicely to the normal range. Normally, our pancreas adjusts to the amount of food we eat, releasing just the right amount of insulin.

So just like when you budget your money at home—so much for your mortgage, heat, and electricity; so much for your weekly groceries and car insurance; and then so much for emergencies—people with diabetes need to budget their insulin the same way. They must have a basal amount of insulin to cover our needs when we're not eating anything, we need insulin to control our meals, and we need some insulin to bring our blood sugars down to normal if they suddenly spike.

Two Canadian physicians, Drs. Frederick Banting and John MacLeod, discovered insulin in 1921. When they injected the first patients, it lasted for only a few minutes, just like the insulin that our body makes. To make this miraculous treatment practical, the insulin molecule had to be modified. Researchers discovered that when mixed with zinc, a number of insulin molecules formed a crystal structure; and when injected into the skin, this crystal structure was absorbed slowly, so that the insulin lasted longer. The amount of zinc in the insulin solution affected the absorption rate. The very first short-acting and long-acting insulins were relatively unstable and unpredictable, and if we tried mixing them together, we ended up with something in between, like mixing orange juice with pineapple juice to get orange-pineapple juice. When mixing insulins, though, we want a combination like oil and water, where the two components retain their characteristics.

A major advance was made in 1936 when *NPH (neutral protamine Hagedorn)* insulin was developed in Denmark. This insulin was relatively stable and didn't change when mixed with other insulins. NPH lasted for about 14 hours and peaked in about 6 to 8 hours. When mixed with the fast-acting insulins, it remained slow acting.

You may be wondering why we relied on beef insulin and pork insulin for so many years. If we were predominantly a fish-eating culture, we probably would have had to develop fish insulin. But we eat so much beef and pork, and the meat-packing industry revolves around these meats. Pancreases from these animals became a great source of insulin once a method of purification was perfected. As more and more people throughout the world developed diabetes, a shortage of insulin became foreseeable. We had a limited supply of beef and pork pancreases, and this meant a potential crisis in the making—not unlike the oil crisis today, where you have a limited supply and increasing demand.

But thanks to advances following the discovery of the gene for insulin in 1978, we began making genetically engineered human insulin by injecting that gene into special bacteria that could multiply very rapidly and become a virtual insulin factory. This *recombinant DNA* insulin was identical to human insulin but had to be purified very carefully to avoid any bacterial proteins in the injection.

The pharmaceutical company Eli Lilly received the first license to produce biosynthetic human insulin, called Humulin. Subsequently, Novo Nordisk in Europe also synthesized human insulin, but it relied on yeast organisms instead of bacteria for cloning. The potential insulin shortage was averted. NPH insulin was the first relatively stable basal, or long-acting, insulin. The human NPH insulin generally had to be given twice a day. It was long acting, for sure, but wasn't quite the steady, flat level expected of a true basal insulin. NPH insulin is a *suspension,* and one must make sure that it is uniformly cloudy prior to injection.

Around 2001, a new era in insulin began with the development of glargine (Lantus), an insulin analog that had very slow-absorbing characteristics. Glargine lasts from 20 to 24 hours in most people. Glargine is a soluble solution of insulin, which doesn't have to be shaken. When injected under the skin, the insulin precipitates and is absorbed slowly. Imagine a slowly melting snowball.

More recently, another long-acting insulin analog has become available: detemir (Levemir). This insulin is attached to a fatty acid. When injected, it binds to the protein albumin. The insulin is then slowly released by the albumin, prolonging the action. At low doses (less than 20 to 30 units per injection), it is similar to NPH in duration, but at higher doses, it may last up to 24 hours.

Inhaled insulins, as well as, other innovations in insulin therapy are being actively pursued.

Practical Tips for Injecting Insulin

Injecting insulin is like dancing, where one partner typically leads and the other follows. When you are using insulin, the hormone becomes the lead, and your food intake follows.

Insulin is available in either vials or in pen devices.

Pens

Insulin pens come in two forms: disposable or for use with replacement cartridges.

A needle tip can be screwed onto the cartridge; then you simply dial the pen cap to the number of units needed. Some pens for children can dispense even half units (in other words, 2 units, 2.5 units, 3 units, 3.5 units, and so forth).

With a pen, the dose is likely to be more accurate. And since the needle tip itself doesn't have to go through the rubber seal of the insulin cartridge, it is not blunted, and the injection tends to be less painful.

One disadvantage to pen injections is that if you are taking two types of insulin, you will need to use two separate pens. The device may also be limited in the amount of insulin that can be given with any single injection. If you're taking a large amount of insulin, you may need to split it up into two injections.

Syringes

The traditional method of injecting insulin has been to insert a needle-tipped syringe into the vial, withdrew the insulin, and inject it. The syringe has unit markings and can come in various sizes, from 30 units to 50 units (0.5 cc) or 100 units (1 cc). Syringes also come with thin or thinner needles and in different lengths.

(Continued on next page)

Injecting Insulin Using a Syringe

1. First, pull the plunger of the syringe to the number of units you need.

2. Wipe the top of the insulin vial and place the needle through the vial's rubber (latex) seal.

3. Press the plunger so that so many units of air are injected into the vial.

4. Then turn the vial upside down and *slowly* pull the plunger back to the number of units needed. Don't pull back too fast, or you will have small air bubbles in the insulin.

5. Once you have the right amount of insulin, remove the syringe from the vial.

6. Grasp some skin (in your stomach area, your upper arms, or your thighs) between your fingers and wipe with an alcohol swab.

7. Hold the syringe like you would hold a pencil.

8. Push the needle into the skin, using a quick one-step motion. Doing this slowly is actually more likely to cause pain.

9. Then push the plunger down slowly until all the insulin has been injected. I suggest counting from one to five, or one to seven.

10. Remove the syringe. You may wish to press an alcohol swab against the skin for a few seconds.

11. To dispose of the syringe, place it in a used plastic bleach bottle that can be tightly sealed.

For intermediate-acting (NPH) insulin, it is important to roll the vial 10 to 12 times to ensure that the insulin is uniformly suspended. Do not shake the vial, since that just creates air bubbles and may lead to an incorrect dose.

If You're Taking Two Kinds of Insulin

Intermediate-acting insulin comes as a cloudy suspension, whereas shorter-acting insulins (regular, lispro, aspart, and glulisine) are all clear. However, the long-acting insulins glargine and detemir are also clear solutions. Although you can mix NPH insulin with the shorter-acting types, never mix glargine or detemir with other insulins in the same syringe.

If You're Taking 40 Units of NPH and 15 Units of Regular Insulin

1. Prepare the vials of insulin.

2. Draw 55 units of air into the syringe.

3. Inject 40 units of air into the cloudy NPH vial.

4. Remove the syringe from the vial.

5. Inject 15 units of air into the regular insulin vial.

6. Withdraw 15 units of insulin into the syringe.

7. Remove the syringe from the regular insulin vial.

8. Now put the syringe into the cloudy NPH vial *without pushing the plunger.*

9. Withdraw 40 units of cloudy insulin into the syringe.

10. Remove the syringe from the vial.

Following these steps will prevent your contaminating the clear insulin vial with the cloudy insulin.

Some insulins come premixed, with 70 percent NPH and 30 percent short-acting insulin, or 50 percent NPH and 50 percent short-acting insulin. These insulins are convenient for folks who are on relatively stable doses of intermediate and short-acting insulins.

(Continued on next page)

Storing Your Insulin

Insulin should generally be stored in the refrigerator but never in the freezer. At room temperature, insulin can be kept for approximately a month. If the insulin is supposed to be clear but appears cloudy, discard it. Avoid storing insulin next to a radiator or in direct sunlight.

When traveling, try to keep your insulin in your hand luggage. You never know the extreme temperatures to which your checked baggage may be exposed. If your diabetes supplies are in their original package, you should have minimal problems with airport security.

Injection Sites

Rotate your injection sites. The stomach is the most consistent site for insulin absorption. Absorption in the arms and legs can be increased by exercise, so if you're active during the day, you could use the stomach for the daytime injections and the arms or legs for the evening, for more consistent insulin absorption.

Basal-Bolus Regimen

A *basal-bolus regimen* (consisting of a basal insulin plus *boluses* to cover your meals) is almost like a poor man's insulin pump therapy. Obviously it's not as sophisticated, but the principle of monitoring your sugar levels and adjusting your insulin doses daily is applied in both types of insulin programs. Both put the person with the diabetes in charge.

Insulin Pumps

Insulin pumps have evolved from the size of backpacks to highly reliable credit card–size instruments. With the use of nanotechnology, the pumps will no doubt get smaller. They are used primarily by men and women with type 1 diabetes but, conceivably, anyone taking insulin could use one. The pumps offer the greatest flexibility of lifestyle but currently depend upon the patient to monitor his or her sugars at least four times a day and to instruct the pump what to do with the insulin delivery. This is called an open-ended loop system.

Choosing an insulin pump is a little like choosing a car. You have to consider how tech savvy you are, what features you need, and what kind of service the manufacturer provides. Of course, you will also need to check with your insurance carrier to find out what coverage, if any, your policy provides. For some comparison information, you may want to visit DiabetesNet.com at *www.diabetesnet.com/diabetes_technology/insulin_pump_models.php.*

GLP-1 analogs (exenatide). Earlier you learned about the incretin hormones GLP-1 and GIP, which act on the pancreas to release more insulin into the circulation. You also learned about the nasty DPP-4 enzymes that cut short incretins' effect. An injectable medication called exenatide (Byetta) prevents DPP-4 from carrying out its dirty work. It's not a DPP-4 blocker, though; the drug boasts the positive properties of GLP-1 but is different enough that it resists the enzymes' efforts to break it down.

Exenatide, available as a twice-a-day injection, is available in a pen device very similar to an insulin pen, with 30 days' worth of doses. Stomach-related side effects have been reported early in the course of therapy, but these usually fade with time. The treatment also appears to lower blood sugar levels effectively and may contribute to weight loss as well. Currently there is clinical research to develop a long-acting preparation that can be given once daily, or once a week, or perhaps even once a month.

Conclusion: The Art of Medicine

Science-fiction writers and futurists have long predicted that computers will replace physicians. However, when I see the list of drugs that can be used for type 2 diabetes, and all of potential precautions and contraindications, and the various patient characteristics, clearly there is more need than ever for thorough, compassionate diabetes caregivers to find the right drug for the right person at the right time.

The best is yet to come.

You may want to visit these websites for complete, reader-friendly information on any of these medications: PDRHealth (*www.pdrhealth.com/home/home.aspx*); Drugs.com (*www.drugs.com*).

Chapter 10

The Future of Diabetes Treatment

I tell my patients not to read medical textbooks to learn about their own diabetes story. Textbooks usually tell you what happened to diabetes patients 15 to 20 years ago, because it often takes that length of time for new theories and treatments to filter down to the public. It's true that with the advent of the Internet, news of developments can reach people more quickly. However, don't jump on the latest fad in clinical care without it being rigorously tested first. Discuss your case with your team of physicians, and weigh the risks and benefits before you decide to try any new medication or technology.

Living with diabetes is like fighting a war: We must be ever vigilant if we are to win. And we want to win. But there are many factors working against us, many of them controllable but unfortunately neglected by us.

Some "Wake-up" Facts about the Future of Diabetes

- Despite advances in medications, diabetes is up 50 percent in the United States in the past decade. One in three Americans born in 2000 will develop diabetes.

- One-third of those with diabetes are undiagnosed. An additional 41 million have prediabetic dysmetabolic syndrome. One-third of those will develop diabetes, but up to 80 percent of those 41 million may die prematurely from heart attacks and strokes.

- The full impact of diabetes is masked by deaths recorded due to other causes (such as heart attacks and strokes) that are, in fact, diabetes related.

- The onset age of diabetes is lowering with each generation; the disease is now appearing in significant numbers of teens.

- Diabetes rates are expected to grow in parallel with economic advances made in developing nations. Within the next 20 years, India and China will experience an explosion of diabetes and related illnesses, with which their medical infrastructures will probably be unable to cope.

- The economic impact of diabetes in the U.S. in 2007 was $174 billion ($116 billion in direct costs, $58 billion indirectly). Millions of Americans are underinsured, which means that the costs will be spread to *all* consumers.

These statistics are daunting and certainly challenging. Nevertheless, there are a lot of exciting advances happening in the field of diabetes, which means that our methods of winning the war are expanding every day. Here are just a few new tools that we hope to have at our regular disposal soon.

Continuous Glucose Sensing

Due to our own disinclinations, cost, and technology, we can check our blood sugars only a limited number of times per day. It's a little like the TV game show *Wheel of Fortune*. We can see some of the letters, but we can't tell the actual phrase. Wouldn't it be helpful to know how our sugars are doing from minute to minute? Then we'd be able to get a more complete picture of our diabetes control.

With the help of a small probe inserted into the fat under the skin of your stomach, there are several new technologies that can document your sugars several hundred times a day for three to seven days. This may not be necessary for everyone, nor is it necessary every day. However, it does appear that the patients who are privy to this information and act upon it can improve their diabetes control significantly.

This technology will develop quickly, and no doubt it will be married to an insulin pump, eventually leading to a closed-loop system. With this type of advance, it is hoped that the pump will automatically adjust the insulin rate based on the sugar results. The person with diabetes would no longer have to calculate exactly how much insulin to take.

Once this is perfected, we may truly be able to achieve tight glucose control safely.

Islet Cell Transplantation

The pancreas contains cells that secrete digestive juices to help process fat, protein, and carbohydrates; beta cells, which manufacture insulin; and cells that make other hormones. Over the years, researchers have tried to separate the beta cells from pancreatic tissue, with the idea of administering them to someone with diabetes and curing that person. The cells could be injected into the liver to make insulin when the sugar level rises to a certain degree. However, anytime that you introduce cells or tissue from another body, the recipient's defense system tries to eradicate it. To prevent *rejection,* patients are given medications to suppress their immune response. In the past, the antirejection drugs needed to protect transplanted islet cells were extremely powerful. Not only that, but they were prone to actually *causing* diabetes. Fortunately, recent improvements to the medications have made them more tolerable for patients, and so the islet cells are able to continue their work.

However: In order for us to harvest enough pancreatic beta cells to benefit one patient with type I diabetes, we typically need two donor organs, although those numbers are improving. Because there is a shortage of pancreases for people with type 1 diabetes, and because many patients could benefit from a pancreas transplant or a combined pancreas-kidney transplant (discussed below), using two pancreases to help one person is seen as an inefficient use of the organs. What's really important is that we're learning a tremendous amount about how beta cells and islet cells work and how they can be protected.

Stem Cell Research

There have been a lot of exciting scientific findings regarding stem cells, as well as some negative commentary on the issue. Stem cells are the "Adam and Eve" of cells. There are adult stem cells and embryonic stem cells, but these are essentially the same and usually reside in our bone marrow. Scientists are investigating how stem cells can be coaxed to develop into specialized cells, like those in your immune system, or brain cells that could treat Parkinson's disease, or heart cells to assist a dying heart—or beta cells to help someone with diabetes.

That sounds very simple, but as the old saying goes, "There's many a slip between the cup and the lip." Take beta cells, for instance: Normally, they respond to small changes in blood sugar levels by releasing insulin into the bloodstream, the right amount at the right time. That ostensibly simple process requires beta cells to recognize sugar molecules and to accurately tell whether their numbers are rising or falling and to what level. Next, it needs to produce just the right amount of insulin to have an effect, then turn off the insulin when the sugar level is appropriate. This gets very complicated. You can imagine the controls that are needed so that someone receiving a stem cell transplant could be secure in knowing that accidents will not happen. You don't want the beta cell to suddenly make too much insulin or to not recognize high blood sugar levels. In order to be practical, stem cell transplants would have to be 100 percent reliable. Many realists in the stem cell research arena feel that it may be 20 years or more before stem cells are available for patients with type 1 diabetes. That may seem like a long time, but bear in mind that insulin was discovered only about 90 years ago.

Another potential approach is to take cells from a pig or a monkey, for example, and by putting in the right genes and controls, make animal beta cells that function and look like human beta cells. This may be one way to avoid some of the ethical issues that people are worried about in respect to stem cell research.

Pharmacogenomics

Our dilemma as we move to the future is knowing that not every drug will help every person. Most people receiving a medication will benefit, but a small percentage may develop complications from that medication, leading to unfortunate tragedies.

But should we throw the baby out with the bath water? Should we take a drug off the market and make it inaccessible to the vast majority of patients who might benefit from the medication? The answer may lie in a rapidly growing field called pharmacogenomics: the ability to identify individuals who might benefit from a certain medication, as well as those who could be harmed by it. In other words, before prescribing Drug A to "Joe," his physician would be able to accurately assess its benefits and risks specifically for Joe.

If the benefit-versus-risk ratio is a little heavy on risk, then perhaps there's an alternative medication that would be just as helpful but less likely to produce side effects. This type of individualized treatment is already being used with some forms of cancer chemotherapy. So in the future, we'll be able to take a drop of your blood, and by analyzing your genes, we'll know which medication will be the most effective and safest for you.

Transplantation Technology

When I was in medical school in the late 1970s, people with diabetes and kidney failure were often not even considered for a kidney transplant. That's changed dramatically. It used to be that transplant recipients had to be placed on powerful immunosuppressive therapies, including high doses of corticosteroids. This increased the likelihood of infections, poorer diabetes control, and a greater chance of developing certain tumors. Today we have safer yet equally effective steroid-sparing therapies, which have opened the doors to transplantation for men and women with diabetes.

The most common transplant procedure is a kidney transplant, typically from a living donor or a cadaver donor.

The technique for pancreas transplantation has improved steadily over the past 30 years. Since a kidney transplant patient requires antirejection drugs, it was natural to think about the possibility of transplanting the pancreas at the same time. SPK (simultaneous pancreas after kidney) has become increasingly popular. Thus, if you have type 1 diabetes *and* end-stage renal failure, transplanting both the pancreas and kidney may have many benefits: cured diabetes,

Tip

Don't forget to sign the organ donor consent form on the back of your driver's license. Each year, we have far more folks on the waiting list than the number of organs available. Who knows: One day *your* life might be saved because someone else signed the back of his or her license.

better protection of the new kidney, and improved quality of life. Some patients may have adequate kidney function but have brittle diabetes, marked by wildly swinging sugar levels. These individuals could also benefit from a pancreas transplant. Since these procedures are complicated and expensive, all transplant programs carefully screen both donors and recipients to ensure the best success rate.

Michael's Story

After living for nearly 30 years with type 1 diabetes, Michael Fisher was close to death. And he almost didn't care anymore, because the 44-year-old was feeling like a 94-year-old. Truth be told, most people who live to 94 are in much better shape than Michael was. But then he had an operation that saved his life, changed his way of thinking, and made him 44 years old again.

I started giving myself insulin shots when I was thirteen, in 1970, right after I was diagnosed with diabetes. And I tested my blood every day, many times a day. They've made tons of progress since then; like, you couldn't test your blood sugar without some huge machine, but now there's a little monitor. Eventually I was taking about twenty-five to thirty blood tests a day because my blood sugar got so wildly out of control.

I played hockey, skied, and rode skateboards when I was younger. Playing hockey, I'd always have glucose with me. I was a goaltender, and during practice I was allowed to keep grapefruit juice with sugar on the back of the net, and I'd sip it every now and then. Back then, you took one shot and prayed that your blood sugar stayed under control. Then they changed that to one shot of half long-acting and half short-acting insulin. Over the years, that kept changing.

My mother never let us eat sweets when we were growing up. We were never allowed to have white bread; we always had to have some dull-tasting whole wheat bread, which we like now, but back then, you know, the neighbors had white bread, but we had this brown stuff. And we were never allowed to have cookies or chocolate, so for me it was no big deal not to have sweets.

I went to college for two years. In my twenties, I was giving myself more and more shots of insulin, more times per day. I was still very active—skiing, rollerblading, playing hockey, skateboarding. Back then, my biggest problem was low blood sugar, not high, because I'd forget to eat, and I'd be doing all this exercise and stuff. Back then, you took two shots a day, and it wore off by the end of the day, so I had to remember to eat, as opposed to forcing myself to not eat.

At first, taking insulin wasn't so bad. I'd take one shot a day. Then, as I got older, I went to two shots a day.

When I was about thirty, I started bringing at least four syringes a day. And at thirty-five, I'd bring this huge glucagon-shot kit that had a needle about the size of a telephone pole; when there was nothing I could do to pull out of a low blood sugar, I'd have to jam this thing into my leg, and it left a gigantic bruise. But it was the only thing that could pull me out of it. I actually wore a fanny pack. Every morning I'd pack a fanny pack with seven syringes and my glucose monitor.

• • • Fast Fact • • •

Glucagon kits have improved over the years.
It's not critical which part of the body you inject,
as long as it gets below the skin. You should
see an improvement in 10 to 15 minutes.

• • •

Sometime in my thirties, I stopped being able to control my blood sugar. I didn't realize it then, but doctors later figured out that nerve damage was causing my intestines to not function properly. So when I ate, my food often just sat there. Up until then, I'd had no problem other than low blood sugar, but I started driving a lot for work, and sitting in that car was probably the worst thing I could do. I'd drive for an hour, get out and do some work, and then drive to another place and do some work.

It was the constant nerve damage that really made me start to go downhill, because a lot of times I'd eat food, and my blood sugar would crash anyway because my food wasn't digesting. The next morning, I'd get up and puke my guts out because it was just sitting there rotting in my stomach. Or my blood sugar would be seventy, and then, an hour later, without eating anything, it would be four hundred because my food suddenly started digesting, even though I hadn't eaten in three or four hours. Fat did that a lot, too. It would make my blood sugar rise at weird times. And that started getting worse and worse and worse, especially combined with not moving around. The doctors tell me the medical term for what I experienced is gastroparesis, or paralysis of the stomach.

I'd never heard of neuropathy until my feet felt like they were on fire, and the doctors told me that was nerve damage. But they didn't realize that my intestines also had nerve damage and weren't working properly. They kept trying to get me to take more and more shots to bring my blood sugar down. I went from the long acting and short acting to multiple short acting. I'd take my blood sugar, and if it was high, I'd take insulin; if it wasn't high, I wouldn't take anything. When I went to restaurants, I'd sit and wait to see my food coming, then run to the bathroom, take my blood sugar, take my insulin, and come back and eat. I was never much of a complainer on stuff like that, so I just kind of figured I was diabetic, and that's why I'm sick and my feet hurt.

But I kept having more and more problems: I started to get almost to the point of passing out from doing any type of exercise. I'd begin to lose consciousness. I used to be able to exercise nonstop, but now I'd start to get woozy and lose my balance and have to sit down. It wasn't so much the low blood sugar but from being out of control: high, low, high, low. I couldn't control it.

I started having seizures because my blood sugar would go from two hundred to thirty within an hour and a half. They say to check into a hospital when you're over four hundred, but that was every day for me; I mean, I was over four hundred every single day.

I lost my driver's license from having multiple seizures and causing a five-car accident. They took my license away permanently. I'd wake up, sometimes on the floor, not knowing what was going on. I remember one time getting up off the floor, and my tongue was bleeding, my glasses were broken in half, and my wife was telling me to lie down. Then I'd have a massive headache for eighteen hours, so bad I couldn't move.

My doctors finally told me I had maybe about two months before I died from the massive seizures I was having. I was having about one a month.

The doctors gave me more and more antiseizure medicine. For instance, a normal amount of antiseizure medication is, maybe, 100 milligrams; a large amount

Red Flag

Brittle diabetes often results from the inability to sense a low blood sugar. If you don't receive the early warning signs, then sugar levels may continue to drop, impairing brain function.

is 200. I was on 630 milligrams of Dilantin. Basically, I sat in a chair for about three years. People brought machines for me to fix, and a couple times my brother took me somewhere to work on a machine. I always thought that tomorrow I'd be better. But I still had seizures, even with the massive amounts of medication. And the medication made me a zombie. I was like a ninety-four-year-old invalid.

I missed about four or five years of my life from being on antiseizure medication, which is like being on heroin or something. I had to quit reading books because I couldn't remember what I read an hour ago. I'd stare at the TV, but I didn't really know what I was watching.

Finally, after trying everything, my doctor told me about pancreas transplants and advised that I might want to consider that. At that point, I felt like I had a couple more years to go until I was dead, so I figured, what the heck? I wound up on the waiting list for seventeen or nineteen months. Then about four years ago, I got the pancreas transplant. At that time, it was still fairly new to do a pancreas-only transplant and not a pancreas-kidney transplant.

It worked. I'm not a diabetic anymore. I can eat whatever I want. I don't take any insulin. My hemoglobin A1C has been perfect. I'm skiing again for the first time in years. My vision has even gotten better.

I take a handful of pills every morning and a smaller handful at night. It's very, very odd: From the time I was thirteen to the time I was forty-four, I took insulin. Before, I was supercareful about what I did. I ate at seven, eleven, and seven, plus snacks, every day for all those years. And now if I'm not hungry in the morning, I don't have to eat. But I'm still getting used to sitting at the restaurant table. I still feel like jumping up when I see my food coming. I feel like something's wrong that I'm not packing up my pockets and my fanny pack.

And I still have my old pancreas. The old one does a lot of other things besides creating insulin. It creates enzymes that help break down food. The new pancreas is placed lower down in the abdomen near the kidneys and bladder.

• • • **Fast Fact** • • •

The pancreas has two main components: the part with islets, which release hormones into the bloodstream; and the bigger part with a large number of ducts that release digestive enzymes into the intestine.

• • •

I'm still not working. I don't quite have my strength, and I still have a little fear of driving. I still can't stop thinking I'm going to have a seizure. I have some permanent nerve and muscle damage. But my doctor says I can go back to work, and I can drive again.

Michael's story illustrates that sometimes the progression of diabetes can be very challenging despite a patient's best efforts to control his or her diabetes. However, with lots of perseverance and a little luck, Michael survived admirably.

Ongoing Research

There's a tremendous amount of research on diabetes under way. For men and women with diabetes, the question isn't how to prevent the disease but how to stop its complications. In the preceding chapters, we covered the practical methods to reduce risks. Clinical research is also being conducted using treatments designed to protect the kidneys from damage caused by high blood sugars. Some of these treatments may also benefit people without diabetes, yet who are having similar problems.

Neuropathy isn't a deadly complication, but it can severely affect the quality of a person's life. Wouldn't it be wonderful to be able to regenerate nerve cells so that sensation can return? A great deal of experimentation is going on to revitalize nerves through gene therapy. For heart disease, there's a new investigational medication that acts like a Roto-Rooter by removing cholesterol from the blood vessels.

So the future looks very bright. And anyone who has diabetes today has a chance to rewrite his or her story and provide a more hopeful ending.

Conclusion

We hope that this book has helped you gain an understanding of diabetes; its causes and risk factors, how in some cases it might be prevented, its early signs, its potential complications, and most importantly, how to minimize the risk of these complications through medication and changes in lifestyle.

Armed with this knowledge, you are now empowered to take the necessary steps to prevent or delay the onset of diabetes if you don't have it, or to improve your chances for a long and healthy life if you do.

As you learned from Ben Dexter in the introduction, ignoring the warning signs of diabetes and the risk factors (especially a family history of the disease) and engaging in unhealthy behaviors can send you hurtling down a slope toward heart disease, eye disease, kidney disease, and nervous system damage. It's never too soon to start prevention efforts;

as you now know, young people today are increasingly at risk for diabetes by being obese and sedentary.

If you are diagnosed with diabetes, the importance of maintaining control over the disease cannot be overstated. Maintaining control will require some time and effort but will pay off in the long run. Here's your checklist of steps to take:

- Monitor your glucose regularly.

- Have your blood pressure and cholesterol levels checked and controlled if they're high.

- Undergo annual eye examinations.

- Have your urine checked for albumin every 6 to 12 months.

- Inspect your feet daily.

- Control your weight.

- Have regular dental checkups.

- Eat a healthy diet.

- For general health, it's also a good idea to avoid alcohol and tobacco and to receive appropriate vaccinations.

If you are on insulin therapy, your doctor has prescribed a regimen to achieve optimum control of your diabetes, which will reduce your chance of developing microvascular disease, especially retinopathy, or slow its progressions. Insulin regimens are chosen to mimic the normal insulin secretion pattern by the pancreas, but they will need to be fine-tuned based on your activity levels and any problems that you might be having with hypoglycemia.

The value of strict diabetes management has been proven without a doubt. A clinical study of more nearly 1,500 patients with type 1 diabetes, called the Diabetes Control and Complications Trial (DCCT), demonstrated that intensive therapy (checking blood glucose at least four times a day and taking four daily insulin injections or using an insulin pump) resulted in a much lower risk of eye disease, diabetic kidney disease, and nerve damage than did less frequent blood glucose checks and insulin injections. When the patients in DCCT were followed for nearly two decades, those who were originally assigned to intensive control had a much lower risk of cardiovascular disease events than the patients who were on less strict glycemic control. The findings from this study have tremendous implications because people with type 1 diabetes face ten times the risk of cardiovascular disease than people who don't have diabetes.

Remember that vascular disease may already be present by the time a person is diagnosed with type 2 diabetes, so a sense of urgency in preventing further damage to the blood vessels is important. Knowing your targets for your blood sugar, hemoglobin A1C (the test to indicate your three-month average of glucose control), cholesterol, and blood pressure will go a long way toward reducing your risk of heart attacks and strokes.

Moreover, keeping your blood sugar between 100 mg/dl and 120 mg/dl is an essential goal, but realize that it may cause occasional episodes of hypoglycemia, which can be managed effectively through diet. Hypoglycemic episodes may be prevented by being consistent with your diet, activity, and use of medications. Also strive to keep your hemoglobin A1C level at 6.5 percent or lower. An optimal blood pressure for a person with diabetes is less than 130/80 mmHg. For your LDL cholesterol—the bad cholesterol—the level should be less than 100 mg/dl, and maybe even less than 80 mg/dl, depending on your other risk factors. Your HDL cholesterol, the good cholesterol, should be more than 55 mg/dl if you're a woman and more than 45 mg/dl if you're a man. An additional lipid target is a fasting triglyceride level of less than 150 mg/dl. Remember that blood sugars that are consistently above 250 or 300 mg/dl signal the need to have your urine checked for ketones, as ketoacidosis may develop.

Some factors that will affect your risk of hypoglycemia include not only your activity level but missed meals, unusually small meals, insulin dosage, and changing your insulin injection site. Your physician will regularly review your blood glucose, insulin dose, and prior experiences with hypoglycemia to limit the risk of hypoglycemia.

Because of the various organs and blood vessels that might be affected by diabetes, and the multiple components of prevention and treatment, having a team of health care providers to help you manage the disease is optimal. You may benefit from consulting with a nutritionist for help in implementing appropriate dietary choices to better manage your diabetes and improve your overall health.

As we saw with Jason Johnson in chapter 5, a positive attitude, a supportive family, and a commitment to taking control of his disease enabled him to thrive in the major leagues. As Jason related, blood sugar testing has become much more convenient, and his treatment has been simplified with an insulin pump. And we see that since he got his pump, Jason remains vigilant with his testing and blood sugar control to "avoid any complications later in life." Jason serves as a great example of someone taking charge of his diabetes. The same is true of Jenny Asher's son Jim, from chapter 6, who got into a routine of managing his disease early in life, and also opted for the freedom of an insulin pump. So did Lisa Linder, from chapter 8, who has no kidney damage and only minimal eye problems 40 years after being diagnosed with type 1 diabetes. Lisa's success stems from her commitment to routine doctor visits, frequent testing of her blood sugar, and her persistence in staying on her prescribed medications.

Hopefully, the stories of the people featured in this book will inspire you to make the wise choices that will give you the best opportunity to lead a long, happy, and productive life. It's in your power! The choice is yours.

Acknowledgments

I wish to thank my grandparents, parents, my wife, Lalitha and children, Pranav, Suparna, Vishal and Pavitra, for their inspiration and support.

Many thanks to all my colleagues at the Cleveland Clinic who strive daily for excellence and expect excellence from each other.

I wish to thank Susan Iannicca, CNP, RD, CDE, who helped me with the chapter on nutrition. And I am grateful to the many patients who shared their stories for this book.

I also want to thank all those that have allowed me to take part in their diabetes care. As they continue to teach me beyond any textbooks, I truly respect how they respond to the daily challenges.

Appendix 1

One Family's Story: The Monks

How a Family Diagnosed with Diabetes Lives to Support One Another

The Monk family—father Alvin, a retired government worker; mother Seville, a retired nurse; and their daughter, Simone, a PhD in education—were all diagnosed with diabetes as adults. Their candid conversation reveals three different attitudes toward and approaches to handling the disease. Their experience, I think, highlights many of the issues discussed in this book.

Here is the Monks' story:

Alvin: I found out I had diabetes in 1980, when I was fifty-one. I had a little car accident, and they discovered in the emergency room that I had diabetes. I think my sugar may have been over five hundred. There were some symptoms that I didn't know were symptoms at the time. I had a hunger for chocolate cake, sweets, all types of sweets. I got to the place where I'd be on my way to work and I'd stop off at doughnut shop and get a doughnut and a loaf cake. I just didn't pay any attention to it. Once, I almost passed out. We went to the park, and I was walking. All of a sudden, I got very dizzy and said, "I better go to the doctor, see what's wrong." But after the incident was over, I forgot it. I ignored it.

There's a history of diabetes in my family, as far as my grandfather. He lost both legs. I think I was twelve or thirteen years old then. Grandma would always get after him, but she'd continue to cook things that weren't good for him. I don't know if my mother had diabetes or not, but she always had a problem with her weight. I have three sisters and one brother, and out of the five of us, four are diabetics.

I have to use ointment and creams, like an antifungal cream on my feet. If I don't, the germs will set in. I have to examine my feet every night. I can't go on the floor without shoes on.

You just have to do what's right. When I found out I had diabetes, I absolutely cried, because I didn't want it. It was a hard thing for me to take; I remembered my grandfather. I want to live longer. I feel that I'm entitled to live past one hundred if I want to. So whatever the doctor has given me to do, I'll do it, and it's no problem for me, because I know if I don't—hey, I'm gone tomorrow.

Sometimes I slip a little, with a piece of chocolate cake or something like that, but it's not as much as I used to do. Maybe a slice and that's it, not half a cake. I don't do those things anymore.

Seville: I was fifty-six when I was diagnosed with diabetes in 1986. All of a sudden, one night I was really, really thirsty. I drank so much water and juice, I thought I was having a cold. I didn't want to think of diabetes. I think if I'd kept my weight down I wouldn't have gotten it, because all of a sudden I gained about seventy, eighty pounds, and I'd never carried this much weight before. So I went to the hospital. My glucose reading was nine hundred. Everything was so blurry. I lost my vision for about three or four days. So they put me on insulin three times a day. I did everything they asked me to do, as far as following my diet and stuff.

• • • *Fast Fact* • • •

It's not unusual to have an extremely high blood sugar level at diagnosis and to need insulin temporarily. Once the patient has been stabilized, lifestyle changes and oral medications may be sufficient to control the diabetes.

• • •

When I first found out I was a diabetic, I was kind of disappointed, because neither my mother nor father were diabetics. I didn't know anyone in my family who was diabetic, so that's why I related mine to weight. But then a strange thing happened: My brother and my first cousins (my mother's sisters' children) all developed diabetes.

I accept it. You get tired quicker than before. I don't have the energy that I used to have to do all the things that I used to do. It takes me longer to do things, but I still do what I've always done. I just pretend that I don't have diabetes sometimes.

I had glaucoma in one eye. My vision out of that eye, as long as the pressure is down, it's very good. I still drive anyplace I want to. I have no problem with my vision, except small print; I have to use a magnifying glass. But as far as distance, I have no problem.

I have no problem with any of my medication. I'm doing all right. Even the Glucophage, I never had a problem with it, I guess, because my dosage is so much lower than my daughter's. I'm on five hundred milligrams twice a day and that's it.

My blood sugar is usually from 80 to about 120. A few weeks ago, I went up to 300 and almost passed out because it's never been like that before. I'd been to several banquets, and they had awfully rich food and I had it.

You really have to be physical to keep that glucose down. My glucose usually runs from about 93 to 110, so I have no problem with that. Dr. Reddy tells me if I lose about ten or fifteen pounds, I could probably come off the pills and control my diabetes by diet. So far I haven't lost the weight.

But it really aggravates me when I see people who won't try to follow their diet, because this is something you have to live with. You have it, and you might as well accept it and do what you're supposed to do. And you really have to exercise when you're a diabetic. That'll keep the sugar down. And sometimes, when it's up high, if you exercise, go for a walk, it'll come down. So I guess I've learned to play with it. You can't sleep all day. Get up and move.

As far as the food goes, you can eat anything you want to as long as you eat everything in moderation. I take my medication every day. I still eat pastries in moderation. That's the way I do it, and I've been doing okay.

One good thing about having diabetes, it teaches you how to eat and live. I know now that I don't have to get up in the morning and eat three and four fried eggs and bacon and sausages and all this kind of thing. During the week, a normal life at home, it's some oatmeal, orange juice, and coffee, or whatever, and I'm gone. I love to eat breakfast; I'm a breakfast person. Being a diabetic, you should eat every two to three, four hours. I'm always snacking on something.

Being a diabetic doesn't really upset me. I've accepted it. That might be my nursing background. Most times, I forget that I'm a diabetic. I don't get depressed. It's just a disease I have to work with. Accept things you can't change and change things that you can. Being a diabetic is not doom. It's not something that's put upon you. You can learn to live with it and live a normal life like anyone else.

Simone: I was totally ignorant of the risk of having diabetic parents. I was working on my dissertation, and I'd get vision problems where there were a lot of circles in my eyes. Yellow circles. And I'd get extreme headaches. I was also on a low-carb diet, and I was losing weight relatively quickly. The day before my fortieth birthday, I went to my doctor for a checkup because I'd lost twenty-five pounds. That's when I was diagnosed as a diabetic. And apparently I'd been one for quite a while.

How a family responds to a disease has a direct correlation to how a person is going to respond to that disease. The best patients are those who are organized and used to routine and aren't rebellious.

It's hard when you're first diagnosed, because you're completely overwhelmed. Doctors are telling you that in order to live longer and live healthy, you have to change your entire lifestyle, that you're going to be in a state of war the rest of your life. I think it's a battle. That's scary, and it can be tiring. And you've got to battle to win and you've got to know that it's long-term, life-term.

Poppy had two cataracts, and he had glaucoma in both eyes. One we didn't catch soon enough. The other one, he had surgery. That's part of the diabetes.

The last time I went to the hospital, I had pancreatitis. That's part of diabetes, too. My parents are blessed. I got diabetes twenty years earlier in my life than they did. These illnesses are trickling down twenty years earlier. If I would've had a child, my child probably would've ended up with the diabetes anywhere between age sixteen and twenty-four.

And the Glucophage has side effects. At first, I had tremendous diarrhea, but I have to let you know that I also have irritable bowel syndrome. Glucophage is tough on the system. The adjustment period, for me, was two to three weeks. It wasn't days; it was *weeks*. I lost five or six pounds in that period.

I need to exercise, too, because I'm also a heart patient. I had a massive heart attack at forty-two and open-heart surgery at forty-three. I'm now fifty. Both sides of my family have heart conditions, and the people that had massive heart attacks didn't live past fifty-two. So I believe I'm doing well and believe I'll make it way past fifty-two. Right now, I'm concerned, and I know I have to watch my kidneys, because I know there's a little protein in the urine.

One of the reasons why I'm not exercising—and this isn't an excuse, it's a fact—I have fibromyalgia. I'm in pain every day, head to toe, to the point that sometimes the bottom of my feet, if I touch the ground, it's painful.

> **Tip**
>
> Exercise has to be individualized. If joint pain is an issue, sometimes water aerobics may be the answer. Or tai chi or yoga.

My problem is also night eating, so you have to figure out something that's going to hold you over so that you can make it without snacking on something at eleven and midnight.

It's hard to follow all the diet rules, though. I think I'm a pretty intelligent person, but I've gone to the dietitian four times, and I don't get it. I remember for maybe a few days, a week, and they give you everything all written out. And I can't remember how to do it, how to make your whole week.

I find diabetes extremely debilitating. The meds I'm supposed to be on right now are Amaryl, 20 milligrams twice a day, and Glucophage, 850 milligrams twice a day. Well, the truth of the matter is that I'm self-employed, and I'm not making enough to stay on my meds all the time. There's no help for people who make *some* money. If you have no money, they *might* help you. So that's where I am.

Do I find diabetes controllable? No. It's something that you can get control of, but it will always be with you, and that troubles me. The only solace or hope I have is that I can help young people—to help them not walk the path that I'm walking. I sit and watch kids in all kinds of schools and churches that are shockingly, overwhelmingly obese, sitting and eating candy all the time.

> ## Tip
>
> It helps to keep a food diary to keep track of your eating habits, because we often eat without realizing it. Also, if you are the shopper in the family, bring home healthy foods, which will make it easier to follow the improved lifestyle.

But how do you motivate people? I don't know. *I have to keep at it myself.* I have to keep taking my medications, try to exercise, eat properly, and do everything else.

You know what changed my entire perspective? Last year Della Reese came to town. She was a spokesperson for the Diabetes Association of Greater Cleveland. One thing she said that I understood very clearly is that no matter how dog-dragging tired you get, you've got to win the war, and that diabetes is the enemy and that you have to have the spirit to fight. Even if you backslide, even if you don't get something right, every day you've got to keep trying, and at the end of the day, thank yourself and thank God that you tried and that you got a little piece done. But don't give up the fight.

That really gave me the extra fire to keep trying. I can do this. It may take me longer than some people. All I can do is just keep trying and keep reaching out to others, so that they don't have to. My students have got to understand that they don't have to go through what I went through. You can slow it down to where it doesn't attack your body and make you worse. You don't lose until you draw your last breath. As long as you're breathing, you have hope. I believe. I'm still in good spirits.

I've lost forty-five pounds, so there's a part of me that expects to continue on. The thing that motivates me the most to stay on this side of the planet is that I have a mission: I don't want children to be like I am. Kids have to have models, and kids also inspire you.

Appendix 2

Know Your Body Mass Index (BMI)

Today, many think that your Body Mass Index (BMI) should be one of the vital signs checked, when you visit a doctor's office. Remember, that you typically get your pulse, blood pressure and maybe your temperature and also your weight. Weight alone doesn't tell us the whole story. However, if we know the height and weight, we can better tell if someone is overweight, obese or normal. The BMI is calculated from knowing the height and weight. What's your BMI? Check the chart!

HEIGHT (IN.)	NORMAL WEIGHT (LB.)						OVERWEIGHT WEIGHT (LB.)					OBESE WEIGHT (LB.)		
BMI (kg/m²)	19	20	21	22	23	24	25	26	27	28	29	30	35	40
58	91	96	100	105	110	115	119	124	129	134	138	143	167	191
59	94	99	104	109	114	119	124	128	133	138	143	148	173	198
60	97	102	107	112	118	123	128	133	138	143	148	153	179	204
61	100	106	111	116	122	127	132	137	143	148	153	158	185	211
62	104	109	115	120	126	131	136	142	147	153	158	164	191	218
63	107	113	118	124	130	135	141	146	152	158	163	169	197	225
64	110	116	122	128	134	140	145	151	157	163	169	174	204	232
65	114	120	126	132	138	144	150	156	162	168	174	180	210	240
66	118	124	130	136	142	148	155	161	167	173	179	186	216	247
67	121	127	134	140	146	153	159	166	172	178	185	191	223	255
68	125	131	138	144	151	158	164	171	177	184	190	197	230	262
69	128	135	142	149	155	162	169	176	182	189	196	203	236	270
70	132	139	146	153	160	167	174	181	188	195	202	207	243	278
71	136	143	150	157	165	172	179	186	193	200	208	215	250	286
72	140	147	154	162	169	177	184	191	199	206	213	221	258	294
73	144	151	159	166	174	182	189	197	204	212	219	227	265	302
74	148	155	163	171	179	186	194	202	210	218	225	233	272	311
75	152	160	168	176	184	192	200	208	216	224	232	240	279	319
76	156	164	172	180	189	197	205	213	221	230	238	246	287	328

Appendix 3

Know Your Estimated Average
Glucose (eAG)

HbA1C %	eAG mg/dl	HbA1C %	eAG mg/dl
6	126	9.6	227
6.2	131	9.8	233
6.4	137	10	239
6.6	143	10.2	244
6.8	148	10.4	250
7	154	10.6	256
7.2	160	10.8	261
7.4	165	11	267
7.6	171	11.2	273
7.8	177	11.4	278
8	183	11.6	284
8.2	188	11.8	289
8.4	194	12	295
8.6	199	12.2	301
8.8	105	12.4	306
9	211	12.6	312
9.2	216	12.8	318
9.4	222	13	323

Remember that if you are not an adult, or pregnant, or belong to a minority group, your estimated Average Glucose level may be a little different from the number in the table.

You should have a hemoglobin A1C test done periodically to let you know what your average sugar levels have been over the previous three months. The eAG is a useful calculation to let you interpret the all-important A1C test.

Remember that if you have a good average but your sugars are fluctuating wildly from day to day, you will obviously know that you are not in good control. The goal should be to get to as low an A1C test (and eAG) as possible, while avoiding extremely high and low blood sugars.

For more information, see the glucose calculator on the American Diabetes Association website, at *http://professional.diabetes.org/glucosecalculator.aspx.*

Appendix 4

Be Informed and Prepared for Checkups

WHAT TO CHECK	HOW OFTEN?	WHAT IS IDEAL?	WHERE ARE YOU NOW?	WHAT'S YOUR GOAL?
A1C (%)	Quarterly	Less than 6.5 or 7		
Blood Pressure (mm Hg)	Always	Less than 130/80		
Cholesterol— LDL (mg/dl)	Yearly	Less than 70		
Dilated Eye exam	Yearly			
Estimated AG (mg/dl)	Quarterly	Less than 140–154		
Foot Exam	Always			
Urine check for albumin (mg/g creatinine)	Yearly	30–300		
Body Mass Index (kg/m^2)	Always	25 or less		
Diabetes Education	Yearly Refresher			
Nutrition	Yearly Refresher			
Sugars before meals (mg/dl)	Regularly	Less than 110		
Sugars after meals (mg/dl)	Regularly	Less than 140		

Whenever you have a diabetes-related medical visit, you should have your blood pressure, weight, eyes, and feet checked. Approximately every three months or so, depending on the stability of your glucose control, you should have your A1C and eAG assessed. This information, along with your own self-monitoring of blood glucose values, will allow you and your health care provider to adjust your treatment plan.

Every year (perhaps around the time of your birthday), you should have your urine checked for protein (albumin); a lipid and cholesterol panel; and a formal eye exam by an eye professional. Occasionally, the eye professional may ask you to come less often.

There's always new research with respect to diabetes and nutrition. It would be helpful to refresh your knowledge from an expert once a year.

Think of your diabetes as your travel partner as you journey through life; a passport that will help keep track of your destinations. You may be interested in the concept of a diabetes passport, which can be viewed at the website of the American Association of Clinical Endocrinologists (*www.aace.com/documents/pdf/DiabetesPassport.pdf*).

Index

About the Author

S. Sethu K. Reddy, MD, MBA, FRCPC, FACP, MACE, is the U.S. scientific director for diabetes and obesity at Merck & Co., a global pharmaceutical company, and immediate past chairman of Endocrinology, Diabetes, and Metabolism at the Cleveland Clinic.

Dr. Reddy earned his MD at the Memorial University of Newfoundland, in Newfoundland, Canada. He completed his fellowship in endocrinology and metabolism at the University of Toronto. His research fellowship in cellular and molecular physiology was conducted at Harvard Medical School's Joslin Diabetes Center in Boston. Prior to joining the Cleveland Clinic, he was associate professor of medicine and biochemistry at Dalhousie University in Halifax, Nova Scotia, Canada. He completed his MBA at Cleveland State University in 2002.

Dr. Reddy's research interests are devoted primarily to clinical endocrinology, including obesity and thyroid disorders, and the epidemiology of diabetes and its complications. He has authored and coauthored more than 120 articles, abstracts, and book chapters concerning these and related topics. He has presented numerous lectures about diabetes management, heart disease, obesity, thyroid disease, and other metabolic disorders at national and international events. He has received more than $1 million in research grants and support for studies related to diabetes and cardiovascular risk factors. He is a fellow of the Royal College of Physicians of Canada, the American College of Physicians, and the American College of Endocrinology. Dr. Reddy is the recipient of several honors and awards, including the Department of Medicine Excellence Award in Teaching. He conceived and developed the nationally recognized Annual Board Review Course, beginning in 1997.

Dr. Reddy has been actively involved in clinically relevant projects with the American Association of Clinical Endocrinologists (AACE) since 1996, including Coding and Reimbursement, Fellowship Training, Optimal Practice of Diabetes Task Force, Endocrine University Program, Socioeconomic Affair, Minority Health Affairs, Clinical Practice Guidelines, and Academic Affairs. He has been elected twice to the National Board of Directors of AACE.

He was also honored with the Florence Nightingale Award by the Cleveland Clinic for Physician Collaboration and as Trustee of the Year in 2005 by the Diabetes Association of Greater Cleveland.

In 2007 he received the distinction of Mastership in the American College of Endocrinology.

This book was completed while Dr. Reddy was Chairman of Endocrinology, Diabetes & Metabolism at the Cleveland Clinic and was recently updated prior to publication.

About the Cleveland Clinic

Cleveland Clinic, located in Cleveland, Ohio, is a not-for-profit multispecialty academic medical center that integrates clinical and hospital care with research and education.

Cleveland Clinic was founded in 1921 by four renowned physicians with a vision of providing outstanding patient care based upon the principles of cooperation, compassion, and innovation. *U.S. News & World Report* consistently names Cleveland Clinic as one of the nation's best hospitals in its annual "America's Best Hospitals" survey. Approximately 1,800 full-time salaried physicians and researchers at Cleveland Clinic and Cleveland Clinic Florida represent more than 100 medical specialties and subspecialties. In 2007 there were 3.5 million outpatient visits to Cleveland Clinic and 50,455 hospital admissions. Patients came for treatment from every state and from more than 80 countries. Cleveland Clinic's website address is *www.clevelandclinic.org.*